FIRST-YEAR NURSE

FIRST-YEAR NURSE

NURSE

Advice on Working with Doctors,
Prioritizing Care, and Time Management

BETH HAWKES, MSN, RN-BC

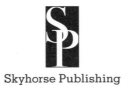

Skyhorse Publishing

Skyhorse Publishing books may be purchased in bulk at special discounts for sales promotion, corporate gifts, fund-raising, or educational purposes. Special editions can also be created to specifications. For details, contact the Special Sales Department, Skyhorse Publishing, 307 West 36th Street, 11th Floor, New York, NY 10018 or info@skyhorsepublishing.com.

Skyhorse® and Skyhorse Publishing® are registered trademarks of Skyhorse Publishing, Inc.®, a Delaware corporation.

Visit our website at www.skyhorsepublishing.com.

10 9 8 7 6 5 4 3

Library of Congress Cataloging-in-Publication Data

Names: Hawkes, Beth, author.
Title: First-year nurse: advice on calling doctors, prioritizing care, and
    time management / Beth Hawkes, MSN, RN-BC.
Description: New York, NY: Skyhorse Publishing, [2020] | Includes
    bibliographical references.
Identifiers: LCCN 2020001165 (print) | LCCN 2020001166 (ebook) | ISBN
    9781510755130 (hardcover) | ISBN 9781510755147 (ebook)
Subjects: LCSH: Nursing—Vocational guidance.
Classification: LCC RT82 .H39 2020 (print) | LCC RT82 (ebook) | DDC
    610.7306/9—dc23
LC record available at https://lccn.loc.gov/2020001165
LC ebook record available at https://lccn.loc.gov/2020001166

Cover design by Mona Lin
Cover images: Getty Images

Print ISBN: 978-1-5107-5513-0
Ebook ISBN: 978-1-5107-5514-7

Printed in China

CONTENTS

NOTE TO READERS: All names referenced in anecdotes or quotations (with the exception of Zach Taylor) have been changed to protect the privacy of all individuals involved. Names used in hypothetical situations do not refer to any specific individual. All advice on administering medical care should only be used as a reference in consideration with standard medical care practices and the rules and regulations for your particular hospital or facility.

LETTER FROM THE AUTHOR

Dear newly licensed nurse,

First of all, thank you for reading my book. I want every nurse to succeed and to love nursing as much as I do.

Use this book like a toolkit. Refer to it as things arise in your first year, and share it with a friend. Hang in there when things are tough and celebrate your successes as they come. Be the best person and best nurse you can be!

Best wishes!
Love,
Nurse Beth

CHAPTER 1

YOU'VE ARRIVED

You made it! You can finally write RN after your name. You've accomplished your dream of becoming a nurse. Now starts your first year. If nursing school was a ride, your first year of nursing will be an even wilder one without the tedious nursing school care plans. Hang on tight for the ride of your life, your first year of nursing.

INSPIRING

Did you know you are admired?

On your way to this point—becoming a newly graduated nurse—you inspired others. Your friends and family tell you they are proud of you, of course, but there are also others around you who respect you for your accomplishment. Others who watched you from a distance and may never tell you. You inspired others to reach their goals, because you accomplished yours.

You most likely look at the experienced nurses around you and admire them for their skills, their calm composure, their ability to get it all done. What you don't know is experienced nurses admire you as well.

What do we see in you? Passion and idealism. The passion to provide the best care and become the best nurse possible. A thirst for knowledge, a hunger to grow. We love your positive energy. We look at each other and nod, "Oh, she's going to be a good nurse" or "We're so lucky our unit got him."

Only your fellow nurses truly understand what it took for you to get to this point. Pre-requisites, applications, worry over being accepted. Early morning clinicals and late night studying. Study groups on Saturday mornings. You're a nurse now, but it came with a cost. You sacrificed time with your family and friends. It was hard and it was exhausting. There were times you questioned your decision. You may have thought about quitting, but you're not a quitter. You dug deep and kept going.

And now nursing school is behind you! Never again will you have to go to the hospital the evening before to create a care plan for the patient you'll be taking care of in the morning. Never again will you agonize over the NCLEX. You'll earn a steady paycheck and it will be wonderful and financially freeing after years of living on a student's budget.

It was not easy. Everyone's path was different, but no matter the path you took, it was uphill. Some of you attended community college and others attended four-year programs. Some of you trained overseas. Some of you are second career nurses. You set your goal and didn't stop until you reached it.

One thing is certain—you're an RN, so you are determined and able to overcome challenges. You have to be smart to be an RN, but being smart alone is not enough. You also have to be determined. No one gets to be an RN unless they really, really want it.

I talked with a newly licensed grad who lived in her car during her last semester and another whose family refused to attend her graduation because they did not approve of her career choice. Regardless, they both were determined to reach their goal. I myself was a single parent with three small children when I attended nursing school.

But now you are here, at the beginning of your new journey and your brand-new career.

Congratulations!

WHAT THEY EXPECT FROM YOU

I was asked this by a newly licensed nurse on Twitter:

> I start on a surgical cardiac step down unit as a new grad RN at the end of this month. My nursing program taught us cardiac basics (emphasis on the basics) so I have been teaching myself the cardiac rhythms, meds. etc. You seem to do a lot with new grad questions so I wanted to see if you had any suggestions on important things a new grad should be proficient in before showing up on a cardiac step down floor.

There are expectations of you, but they are not what you think. You aren't expected to have anything more than basic knowledge, which you have—you passed the NCLEX. It's not an expectation for you to be proficient in anything yet because you are a novice. There is no way to become proficient in nursing practice through book study alone. No one expects you to understand the nuances of ABGs and no one will be disappointed or think less of you because you can't read EKGs.

So many new nurses going for an interview ask me the same question—what should they study up on to make them a better candidate on a particular unit? As a newly licensed nurse you are no more or less qualified than every other newly licensed nurse.

Those of you with a job were not hired because of your expert knowledge. During interviews you were not quizzed on the Krebs cycle in order to find the best candidate, were you? However, you did stand out among the others and you were chosen. Why? They see the nurse you will become. They have invested in you, and planned for you, because they see the potential in you. You were hired because of that potential, and because they believe you'll be a good fit.

So, in answer to the Twitter nurse's question, you are expected to be teachable. You are expected to be on time. You are expected to ask questions and then ask more questions. You are expected to be a safe practitioner and to show initiative.

Your educator has likely oriented many newly licensed nurses and has an educational plan for you. It may involve first taking a Basic Arrhythmia course, then taking ACLS, then becoming stroke certified, or a like plan depending on your unit and specialty.

Here's a tip for those of you who plan to become Nurse Practitioners (NP): Do not expect talking about your future plans to become an NP to be well-received as a newly licensed nurse. If that's your goal, fine, but for now just focus on being a nurse.

Likewise, avoid being a know-it-all. Know-it-alls are especially not appreciated. If you are a know-it-all, you are probably smart. But there are different kinds of smart, and you need to be emotionally and socially smart as well as IQ smart. If you can repress your need to be acknowledged and be smart enough to listen and learn, you can go far. This is a time for listening and learning. Talking about yourself interferes with that.

TRANSITION TO PRACTICE

Maybe you had top grades in school, and perhaps you were even the class president, but now you're starting over. It's exciting and it's uncomfortable and it's why it's called transition to practice.

In school you were insulated from the real working world. You did not carry the phone in clinicals, and you were exempt from many of the duties of a staff RN. You did not have to call doctors, or manage a code, or decide when to call a rapid response team (RRT). You did not delegate to patient care technicians (PCTS) or certified nursing assistants (CNAs). You were protected from overload and you didn't cover another nurse's lunch break or work short staffed.

Most likely you had one or two patients at a time with limited responsibilities. Clinicals typically do not last for eight and twelve hours, so you had a slice of a shift, not an entire shift. You had tasks, but priorities and tasks in nursing school are predictable and linear, whereas priorities and tasks in the working world are constantly shifting.

You are going to be immersed in bridging the sizable gap between nursing school and nursing practice this first year.

In addition to the gap, there's reality shock.

REALITY SHOCK

Know that you will go through stages described as "Reality Shock" by Marlene Kramer (1974). They are all normal. It's part of the process. In her seminal work, Kramer defines the four phases of reality shock as the following:

- Honeymoon phase
- Shock phase
- Recovery phase
- Resolution phase

Honeymoon Phase

The honeymoon phase is just that, the honeymoon, and it's wonderful. Enjoy it. It's that phase when you first start a new job, filled with excitement and anticipation. You have lots of energy and confidence. It's likened to wearing rose-colored glasses, because the reality of the practice setting, with all its inconsistencies and flaws, has not yet sunk in. Everything is pretty in pink and indeed rosy. You love your coworkers, the unit, and the organization. There are no negatives.

It's a good time to introduce yourself to colleagues and doctors, as it's easy to be outgoing and positive. During this stage, you will be establishing relationships with your co-workers and enjoying your new position.

While it's an exciting phase, like all honeymoons, it doesn't last forever.

Shock Phase

The shock phase is when reality sets in. You begin to notice that things are not perfect. You overhear coworkers gossiping in the breakroom. The night shift leaves the computers on wheels unplugged and uncharged. You can't find the bladder scanner because no one puts it back where it belongs. The charge nurse is not especially approachable and takes long breaks.

You're dismayed with aspects of your new job. You may realize that instead of having one preceptor or one primary preceptor and one secondary preceptor as planned, you have several preceptors. You may be disillusioned when you realize the amount of time you have to spend on computer documenting. When reality shock is at its worst, you may wonder if you are on the right unit, in the right facility, or even if nursing is the right profession for you. You may go so far as to question your decision to become a nurse and wonder if you're really suited to this.

Reality shock describes the fairly predictable reactionary process that you undergo when you transition from student nurse to registered nurse and discover that the job is not what you expected. Reality shock is not limited to newly licensed nurses, it takes place when the realities of any new job sets in. Experienced nurses, too, experience reality shock when they transition to a new practice area.

A newly licensed nurse working night shift in ICU noticed that the lab tech was going from patient to patient drawing blood for morning labs without changing her gloves. She was shocked and reported it to her manager, who talked with the lab director. The situation was corrected but she wondered what kind of organization she had gotten herself into. How could people ignore best practice, become so blasé, and put patients at risk? Surely, they were trained properly.

The solution to the shock of transition to practice is biculturalism. It's learning to work successfully in the real world while keeping your high standards.

Biculturalism

"Biculturalism" is the integration of two seemingly conflicting cultures and sets of values. The two cultures are the culture of nursing school and the culture of the practice setting. The two sets of values are the values learned in nursing school and the values of the practice setting.

As an example, in nursing school, you were taught to do comprehensive patient assessments. It can easily take fifteen minutes, if not longer, to perform a head-to-toe patient assessment. But on the nursing unit, you must do your patient assessments in just minutes in order to get everything else done. It's rare that you'll have fifteen minutes of uninterrupted time, much less fifteen minutes for each patient, and all within a couple of hours of coming on shift. So, you are faced with what seems to be opposing values: being thorough versus being quick. In reality, you do not have to give up either. You must learn to become quickly thorough by being laser focused. You learn to focus on the systems with presenting problems. If you have a post-op patient with a hip replacement, your assessment will focus on the wound and mobility. For the neuro and cardiac portions of the assessment, you will spend less time, charting "within defined limits" as your facility allows.

> As a student LPN, Joan was trained to provide what was called "hs care." If you worked evening shift, you were expected to round on your patients, change their pillowcases, and offer them a backrub. Baths included soaking the feet in a basin of water, not just wiping with a cloth. This was easy enough to do with two patients during clinicals and under the eagle eye of the nursing instructor.
>
> On Joan's first shift as an LPN she was assigned eight patients. She was in shock and wondered if there had been a mistake. How was she possibly going to get all that foot care done? Surely if that was the expectation, she should only have three, maybe four patients tops, right? Joan quickly learned to prioritize care, delegate, and let go of some of the good but unrealistic goals she was taught in nursing school.

Recovery and Resolution Phases

Nurses who successfully make it through the shock phase learn not to abandon their ideals but to embrace new ways of getting things done. Nurses who are not able to reconcile the two sets of values end up leaving the job and sometimes the profession.

It's important that you vent your concerns in a positive manner. Make a list of solutions along with your list of problems.

Get involved with your shared governance or unit based council or whatever structure is in place.

> Jan went to work in the medical-surgical (med-surg) unit right after graduation and she was shocked that the only way to change a patient gown was to disconnect the IV tubing, pull the tubing through the sleeve in the patient's gown, and reconnect the two exposed ends of the IV tubing. She couldn't bring herself to do this, because it had been drilled into her in nursing school to never disconnect an IV line unnecessarily due to risk of infection. When she saw nurses casually disconnecting the IV line for every gown change, she was appalled.

What did Jan do? She went to her manager with the problem, and the hospital started ordering patient gowns from another vendor. A vendor who supplied patient gowns with snaps on the sleeves to change IV tubing. Sometimes newly licensed nurses bring a welcome new set of eyes to the unit.

The challenge is to accept the reality of the situation while preserving your ideals. There are nurses around you to help you do this. They've all done it, and you can, too.

NOVICE TO EXPERT

According to Patricia Benner's model of skills acquisition, there are five categories—novice, advanced beginner, proficient, competent, and expert. In this first year, you are practicing as a novice then as an advanced beginner.

As a novice nurse, your tools for practice are the rules you learned in school, called rule-based behavior. It's a necessary first step where you apply rules without context.

You will be in several situations where you know that there are things going on that you just don't fully understand, such as an RRT or a code. It takes time to see the big picture. This is a normal part of your progression. Doctors will give you orders but not explain the rationale behind the orders. You know that you don't understand things the experienced nurses around you do, who seem to have a good grasp on what the doctors are saying or ordering. As soon as possible when something like this happens, ask your preceptor to explain. This is how things will begin to fall into place for you and make sense.

As an advanced beginner, you move from abstract principles to concrete experience. Acquisition of clinical knowledge and skills takes place in sequenced steps.

For example, a child learning to tie their shoes for the first time is a novice at tying shoelaces. They must painstakingly learn one step at a time. Holding one shoelace in their left hand, one shoelace in their right, crossing the right over the left, pulling it under, and so on. Feeling all thumbs. When they are in this stage of learning they must concentrate fully on the task at hand and recall each step in order.

Eventually it becomes easier. With practice the steps are integrated, and they can do it smoothly and with less concentration. The child can tie their shoes quickly and correctly every time.

Eventually they have synthesized the steps so completely that they perform on autopilot. They may not be able to break down the steps to show someone else even if they wanted to. They are at the expert stage.

In nursing, as in many professions, there is a benefit to learning a skill or task so well that one can perform it without thought, as second nature.

It's the same when you learned to ride a bike. Competence and expertise come with time and you can't circumvent or rush the process. Sometimes preceptors forget this and are impatient. There is a saying that you must do things seven times before you remember. Give yourself credit for your progress.

POSER ANXIETY

There may be times when you feel you are outwardly presenting as a nurse but inwardly feel like a poser. You will worry about yourself and your abilities, how others perceive you, that you might miss something, and that your patient might be harmed or, worse yet, die.

It's true that you are confronted with an immense amount of information to process and often without the time to do so. You are expected to jump in during rapidly changing clinical situations. At such times, use the tools of basic safety and call for help. Take a deep breath and focus. Basic safety means assess for airway, breathing, circulation. O2 sats low? Apply oxygen. Get a set of vitals. These are things you can do and are trained to do.

You are genuinely a nurse and you are experiencing what every single nurse before you has experienced. It takes time and it does get better!

What I've learned is that whatever you think or feel, you are not alone. In fact, I started my award-winning blog, nursecode.com, around that concept. You will feel repulsed by some sights and smells—you are not alone. You'll have self-doubt, you'll have deeply gratifying moments, and you'll feel alone at times, but you are not alone.

A time will come when you will know that a patient and you crossed paths for no other reason than destiny so you could help them at that exact moment.

Kati Kleber, known as the Fresh RN, is a renowned nurse influencer, author, and blogger. She wrote the following:

When I graduated from nursing school and passed boards, I was so excited to finally be a nurse. Only, I didn't feel like a nurse. I felt alone. I felt like somehow everyone else knew exactly what they were doing, and I was the only one who didn't belong. I desperately wanted to sit down with an experienced nurse and chat about all of the ins and outs, the cool things to do and the not so cool things to do, and dive into what it's really like at the bedside . . . not what my textbook says . . . what it's really like.

I would have loved to ask that nurse on my unit I admired so much because she seemed to know the answer to everything, was calm and confident, and so smart, if she could meet me for coffee for about four hours every week during my orientation process. But I have a feeling that would have fallen into the "not cool" category, right?

A little much? Yea, probably.

Even though I wanted to do that, I didn't. I stepped out into the nursing wilderness alone and scared, unsure if I'd make it through.

Well, that was back in 2010. Since then, I've worked med-surg, step down, and neurocritical care. I've been a preceptor, mentor, charge nurse, and now I am an educator. Despite all of the experiences all these years later, those feelings of isolation, insecurity, fear, and loneliness are still palpable when I think back to when I was that fresh new nurse. I never forgot them.

Every nurse goes through the same experiences you are going through.

ACCEPT AMBIVALENCE

It can be distressing to learn that nursing and medicine are not black and white. Ambivalence is something you must learn to accept, however uncomfortable, and it makes you a better nurse. In school you were given clearly defined normals and abnormals, but those were without context.

For example, when you take ACLS or Basic Arrhythmia, you learn that ventricular tachycardia (V-tach) is a lethal, wide-complex QRS. Then on the floor a patient has a run of a fast rhythm with a wide QRS complex. You run to the room and he's sitting up eating breakfast and watching TV, blood pressure is fine. The monitor tech prints out a six second strip of the event for you. A cardiologist is rounding, you show him the strip, and you ask his opinion. He says it's a junctional rhythm with aberrant conduction. Later you ask a second cardiologist and he says it's V-tach.

The truth is, they both gave a viable answer with limited information (a six second strip and without an EKG).

There are few absolutes, so keep an open mind. It makes you a better thinker.

Once I had a 45-year-old woman with lupus in ICU who drove herself to the hospital in V-tach. Once there, we kept shocking her, but she kept going back into V-tach. She was put on a Lidocaine drip, then a Pronestyl drip. We did serial EKGs. The whole time, she was awake, so we'd have to sedate her before shocking her each time. Multiple specialists were consulted. Every nurse in ICU came to see because it was so unusual. It didn't fit any of the rules.

So did the fact that she was awake mean she was not in V-tach? Were all the doctors and nurses wrong? Or was this one of those cases that don't follow the textbook?

GIVE YOURSELF ONE YEAR

Don't underestimate the importance of your first year. This is when you bridge the gap from school to practice. From novice to advanced beginner. From dependent to independent. It's estimated it takes one year to feel comfortable.

Commit to this dedicated first year. If you are an ADN planning to get your BSN, wait one year. If you are a BSN going back for graduate school, wait at least one year. It will take all of your mental and emotional energy to learn your role this first year, and if your attention is divided between two goals, both will suffer.

Your focus needs to be completely trained on this first foundational year as you establish your nursing practice.

As a nursing career columnist for allnurses.com, I receive career questions daily. I received an "Ask Nurse Beth" question from a newly licensed nurse asking if she should take a position as a private duty nurse or in a long term care (LTC) facility. She believed that since she graduated, she was ready to be an independent practitioner. In reality, her learning is just starting. I was glad when she took my advice and declined the private duty position.

Any practice setting where you practice alone, such as in home health or private duty, is not recommended for a newly licensed nurse. Likewise, agency work is recommended for nurses with at least two years of experience, and any agency that hires a newly licensed nurse is not reputable. That is because, as an agency nurse, you are expected to hit the ground running with only one to two shifts of orientation.

Whether you landed your dream job in your first choice of specialty or not, most essential skills can be learned in any unit—for example, time management. Be prepared for the fact that your choice of specialty may change. Most nurses will change specialties during their career.

SCRUBS AND SHOES

No longer do you have to wear the poorly fitting, boxy scrubs in colors you detested as a student nurse. There are a lot of great brands out there, and with all the choices you can find the scrubs that are perfect for you and your body type.

The more expensive scrubs cost more for a good reason. The materials are soft and amazing, they last longer, wash well, the color is truer, they are flattering, and they have better design. Better design means they hang better on your body and make you look better. Buy yourself at least one pair of high-end scrubs and you'll see the difference.

Wearing good scrubs means you will look better and feel better. Don't skimp on scrubs or shoes. You're a professional; present yourself as one with quality clothing.

Without going into brand names, there are also many great shoes for nurses out there. You may have already found your go-to shoes while in school. A great way to find the best scrubs and shoes is to look and see what other nurses are wearing. Pay attention to what brands nurses with the same body type as you are wearing and ask them. If you are tall and your length is in your torso, you need scrub tops that are cut a little longer. When you bend over, you want adequate coverage on your backside with no skin exposed. If most of your height is in your legs, you need scrub pants that are cut longer and don't leave you with high waters. Another thing I do when shopping is talk to the store staff and asking "What is your best-selling brand?"

Some local uniform shops have an agreement with local hospitals and offer a discount to nurses with a hospital-issued badge.

IT'S A SMALL WORLD

It may not seem like it to you now, but nursing is a small world. Throughout your career, you will run into nurses and coworkers you worked with at a different time in a different place. You can even end up being the boss of the nurse manager who once hired you for your first job (as is my boss!). Networking starts right away, with your first job.

You will be unforgettable to patients for whom you didn't even know you made a difference and can't even remember. Many times, I've had a patient I didn't recognize stop me out in the community.

Once I had a man stop me on the street and warmly say "Hi! Remember, you took care of my wife." I didn't really remember, and I said "Oh, yes. How is she?" He replied, "Remember, she died. You were her angel." "Oh, right, I'm sorry" (cringe). Not my best moment.

Let's see best how to help you navigate the real world of nursing. This book is to help you bridge the gap between nursing school and nursing, to launch your career. It's to give you some real world tips and tools in your toolbox.

It's practical and informative, two of my core values. I hope you enjoy it and I hope it helps you, my friend.

Keep learning. Becoming a nurse is a journey like no other. It will be extraordinary, I promise. This next year will be amazing. From day one, you will accrue unforgettable stories and memories. You will laugh and you will cry. Expect a roller coaster ride and welcome to the world of nursing.

CHAPTER 2

ORIENTATION EXPECTATIONS

PREPARE FOR YOUR FIRST DAY

It's your first day on the unit! Bring cash in your scrubs pocket and leave your purse securely locked in the trunk of your car. Your badge may not yet be activated or work in the cafeteria right away. You may not have been assigned a locker yet. If you are carrying your phone, slip it in your pocket and make sure it's on mute.

Be on time. In nursing, as in clinicals, being on time means not only clocking in on time but being ready to go without delay. Have two pens in your pocket, a clipboard, belongings in your locker (if you have one), and your mind clear, ready, and focused on the shift ahead.

Before your first day of work, do a dry run. Drive to work at the same time of day you will be working, using the same route and parking close to where you expect to park as an employee. Be sure to time how long it takes you from door to door.

Pay attention to what's available in the nurses' lounge—a refrigerator, a microwave—and note any restrictions on use.

Many nurses choose to bring their own meals to make healthy choices and control what they eat.

Cover your tattoos until you are sure of both the dress code and the culture. The hospital industry as a whole is conservative.

NURSE RESIDENCY PROGRAMS

Nurse Residencies are the gold standard for newly licensed nurses. They ease the transition into clinical practice and are intended to aid in retention for your employer. Your hospital is very interested in keeping you satisfied and retaining you as an employee.

Lasting anywhere from six to twelve months, residency programs help you to develop critical thinking and time management skills, both of which help you succeed in practice.

Typically, you are placed with a preceptor for about twelve weeks, longer in the specialty areas. Nurses in L&D, ED, and ICU may spend eighteen weeks or longer with a preceptor. Every facility is different and time lengths will vary. Either way, as a resident, you are with a preceptor longer than non-residency new hires. You are closely followed by your educator. In some residencies you are also paired with a mentor, who serves as a guide and a support.

If you are lucky enough to get into a residency program, take full advantage of it. Use this as a time to learn while you have full backup.

Classes

Clinical days on the unit are supplemented with educational days in staff development and training. The classes are intended to build on information you received in school and provide information that is facility-specific—for example, a class on surgical and procedural consents and how to complete them.

Other examples include a class on administering blood trans-fusions or a skills lab on chest tubes and drainage. ICU nurses receive a class on IV vasopressors. In addition, you will be given Basic Arrhythmia, ACLS, and PALS if you don't already have them and if they are required for your specialty area.

No Vacations
Don't plan vacations during your residency program.

> Brittany was a newly licensed nurse. It was hard to tell who was happier and prouder, Brittany or her husband. As a secret he planned an elaborate, expensive 2-week cruise to the Mediterranean with a no-refund policy. He presented Brittany with the tickets and she was outwardly pleased but inwardly dismayed. She was now in the position of having to ask for 2 weeks off when she had been told over and over, "There is no time off during the residency."
>
> The last thing Brittany wanted to do was to hurt her husband's feelings. She told him the cruise date would still be in the middle of the residency and he said, "So? You can make it up."

The reason for not allowing time off during the residency is that essential classes are provided, and frequently there are no make-ups. For example, a class that includes a group discussion or small-group role playing cannot be given to one person.

As it turns out, because of the timing and because the residency manager and educator were understanding, they were able to work it out. Brittany went on her Mediterranean cruise.

Project
Many residency programs culminate with a team project—such as a poster presentation—on a performance improvement

topic of your choice. The projects I've seen have been inspiring and informative. I've seen ICU residents institute a hydration station that complied with CDC standards, so the ICU nurses didn't have to go to the break room to drink water. In a different cohort, the telemetry (Tele) residents were instrumental in getting break nurses for their floor in order to maintain safe nurse-patient staffing ratios during break times.

The presentations have become so meaningful and popular at my hospital that they now include a luncheon and are attended by preceptors, managers, and directors. This is because newly licensed nurses are amazing and innovative.

> *Overall, I believe this project was an amazing opportunity to make changes and progress for our patients. It's important for new grads to get this experience because we have not been in the hospital for a long time, so we get to see from a learning experience what we think might work a little better. It's exciting to know as a new graduate we get the same opportunities to make change as the experienced nurses. We possibly can make even more change because we have not been doing a skill or assessment the same way for many years, thus making it easy to mold us into the great nurses we know we can be.*
>
> **—Essence H., new resident**

> *This project allowed me to see more of the big picture that is evidence-based practice, and for that I am grateful.*
>
> **–Anonymous new graduate**

Debriefing

Debriefing is an important part of many residency programs. In debriefing, residents are broken up into small groups, usually eight to ten residents, with a facilitator or a facilitator and co-facilitator. Groups are seated in a circle, and it's a safe place to share challenges and wins, progress and setbacks. The groups are purposefully made up of nurses from different specialties. The reason is to understand that everyone is sharing common experiences, regardless of specialty.

Whether or not your program has debriefing sessions, know that you are not alone. Your peers, newly licensed nurses, are experiencing the same feelings as you, no matter what unit they are in. Becoming a competent practitioner takes time. Do not blame yourself, give yourself grace, and respect the process.

> Lisa was struggling with her preceptor, who criticized her in front of her patients and was overly directive. The preceptor was recognized as being an expert nurse with uncompromisingly high standards, but she was impatient and tough on new hires. Several residents in her debriefing group offered suggestions to Lisa, ranging from going to her educator, her manager, or the program manager, to talking directly to the preceptor herself. Lisa decided to talk to her preceptor herself, and in the group, she rehearsed different approaches and language. Two weeks later, the group met again. Lisa was beaming. "I told her how I felt when she made me look like a student nurse in front of patients. She said she had no idea she came across like that and from her point of view, she was just trying to make me the best nurse I could be. But she actually changed and thanked me for her feedback."

Here's one of my earliest memories as a nurse:

> As a new nurse I was floated to ICU. The patient I was assigned to was critical and was expected to die. He had a Do Not Resuscitate status. Even so, I was instructed to

sit by the bedside and check his vitals every fifteen minutes. At the time, we took manual blood pressures with a stethoscope and blood pressure cuff. I still remember how sore my ears were the next day from taking the earpieces in my stethoscope in and out of my ears every fifteen minutes. He was unresponsive the entire time, and the assignment was tedious. A few hours into the shift, his breathing changed, and then he suddenly took his last, shuddering breath. At least I thought it was his last. It seemed like an entire minute passed and he did it again. An unearthly sounding, gasping breath. This time it was his last. Shocked, I remember looking up and searching around the unit. Everyone appeared normal. I could still see the nurse manager standing in the middle of the unit, nonchalantly chatting with a doctor, coffee cup in hand.

I was in shock and wondered how everyone could be acting normally. Someone just died! Right in front of me. I had never seen a dead person. I had never experienced death whatsoever except for my pet cat. The fact that years later I still recall the feelings and details so vividly tells me I have a certain amount of PTSD around the event. I had no idea what to do or how to feel. I went to the charge nurse and said "My patient just died." They responded, "Okay, you can go back to Tele now and see if they need you. Thanks, Beth!"

So I pushed down my feelings, put on a poker face, and went downstairs to my home unit. I learned that day that that's how I was supposed to respond. To not respond. Or so I thought. But not talking about feelings doesn't work. Talking about feelings is the best way to process them.

I hope you have a debriefing component in your program, but debriefing can be informal or formal. What's most important is to talk with someone. Whatever you are experiencing or feeling is not new—others have experienced and felt the same thing.

Fortunately, I have a husband who I can talk to and debrief with, but even a loving, supportive husband will not always completely understand when it comes to nursing issues. If you are feeling overly stressed, find out from human resources if your facility has an employee assistance program (EAP). EAPs provide anonymous, free or discounted therapy sessions to employees. They can be used for talking about any nature of problem, not just work problems.

PRECEPTOR

The best preceptors love to precept new nurses. They commit to your development and rejoice in your success. I have precepted many new nurses myself and each one of them holds a special place in my heart.

In my hospital, an example of a committed, passionate preceptor is Zach. Weeks ahead of time, Zach prepared for his preceptee and jotted down the following:

Surgical-Telemetry 5N/5E
Q4H vitals, Q4H assessment on tele and on drains/wounds
First thing in AM: vitals, labs, meds, orders, progress note (if time)
Check Kaiser vs Sound group etc. #
- *Five rights of medication administration*
- *PO, IV, IM, SQ, Primary and secondary IV med administration. One hour before and one hour after leeway for ordered timeframe (except stat medications)*

- *Common lab K 3.5–5.0*
- *Mg 1.8+*
- *Hgb > 8*

Assessment/medication pass

Charting thereafter (IView). Acuity and deciding which patient to prioritize

Relieving the monitor tech once the arrhythmia exam is passed (search "basic arrhythmia" in HealthStream catalog for practice 7 video series). What to lookout for.

White wristband for chest pain patients.

Lead orientation for telemetry monitoring

Crash cart locations, clean utility, break room, soiled utility, isolation supplies, nutrition pantry. Central Omnicell vs west/east Omnicell. Patient bins and refrigerated medications. Common unit numbers and passcodes to doors.

K/Mg protocol for low potassium and magnesium levels. Type "combined" when ordering for MD . . . will show up.

ACS (troponins/ekg trend . . . stress test vs angiography) and CVA (NIH scale, NPO until swallow screen, anticoagulants, PT, OT, Speech) measures

SCIP/VTE/Progressive mobility for surgical patients

CHF measures /Amiodarone gtt/Heparin gtt

Zach is going to make sure that his preceptee has the tools and information they need to succeed. Thanks, Zach Taylor, for sharing and allowing me to publish.

You will be assigned at least one preceptor during your orientation. Or you may be assigned one primary preceptor and one back-up preceptor. In reality, you may have more than one or two preceptors. Your preceptor may call in sick one day or even forget to tell you they have a vacation day planned. In that case, the charge nurse will assign another nurse to be your preceptor for that shift. Here's a tip, and let's hope it doesn't happen, but it's possible this other nurse will not appreciate being taken by surprise and may not be particularly gracious in the moment. What I'm saying is, if she rolls her eyes, don't take it personally. It's not about you, it's about not liking being blindsided. She'll warm up to you as the shift goes on.

The real downside is that the new preceptor will not know what you've already done in orientation. It may feel like starting over and having to prove yourself to this new preceptor. It's helpful for you to articulate what you've accomplished thus far, and your goals for the shift. The upside is that every preceptor brings something different to the table, and the person that benefits from the differences in practice is you. You will find that every nurse organizes her day differently. You get to incorporate the pieces that work for you, and by the end of orientation, you will have your own way of practicing nursing.

There are certain things you can expect from your preceptor.

Some hospitals use the "married state" where you and your preceptor are joined at the hip, so to speak. Instead of the traditional model where you and your preceptor split the team of patients, you take all the patients together as a team. The resident performs assessments on all of the patients to start with, then medication administration is added, and so on, until you're managing all of their care, but with your preceptor by your side. In this way you are not left to manage on your own, and your preceptor is always there to coach you.

What if the worst happens and you are left on your own?

Lindsey was in ICU working the third twelve hour shift of her orientation. Her preceptor was also assigned to "buddy" with a nurse who had floated in from another unit. The preceptor was called away to help the float nurse with her patient a few beds away and across the nurses' station. Meanwhile, the GI team came up to do a procedure on Lindsey's patient and started asking Lindsey questions she had no idea how to answer. The GI doctor gave her patient an IV medication. The patient's heart rate immediately went up to 160 and the blood pressure went up to 188. Lindsey had no idea what to do. She called out to her preceptor, who was now busy trying to extubate the float nurse's patient. Her preceptor told her to call the charge nurse, but the charge nurse was in a meeting to plan staffing for the next shift. Fortunately, another experienced ICU nurse stepped in to help Lindsey.

What could have gone differently? When Lindsey's preceptor was leaving to go help another nurse and told Lindsey to remain at the bedside, Lindsey could have spoken up and said, "I'm not comfortable being alone, shall I come with you?"

Protector
One of your preceptor's roles is to be your protector.

Julie was standing in the nursing station and overheard her preceptor talking to another new grad's preceptor. "How's your new grad doing? Mine's amazing. She's really bright and asks lots of good questions, I love that."

Most preceptors take a great deal of pride in helping you grow, and your preceptor has your back. They should talk you up to your colleagues and providers.

In good preceptor-resident relationships, your preceptor is your biggest fan and does everything to help you succeed.

Socializer

Another one of a preceptor's roles is that of socializer. You should expect your preceptor to socialize you to the unit. This means eating meals with you and taking breaks with you. Introducing you to coworkers and doctors. Explaining the mores and culture of your unit. What does it mean if your nurse manager's door is shut? Is it okay to knock and enter, or does it mean don't enter at all? If the nurses on your floor pool their food in the middle of the table, what does that mean? Is it okay to join in? If there's an upcoming potluck, you should be informed that only senior nurse Lisa brings the enchiladas, and they're her specialty. A good preceptor will be by your side as you are integrated into the team.

Evaluator

You should be given regular, meaningful, and constructive feedback. Receiving feedback can be humbling but seeking and receiving feedback on your performance is an expected part of professional development.

Often preceptors neglect to give sufficient feedback. This is a source of distress for new grads who really need to know how they're doing.

FEEDBACK

Feedback is highly important to you, but you may have to prompt your preceptor to get it. If your preceptor is not giving you regular feedback, then you need to ask.

At the end of the shift, ask your preceptor for feedback. Consider establishing a habit of walking out together after your shift to the parking area. This is a good time to debrief about the shift, what went well, and what didn't go so well.

"Can you give me feedback on my performance today?" and "Is there something I should have done differently?" are both good questions to ask.

If your preceptor says, "You're doing good," ask for more specific feedback. Say, "Thank you! What specifically am I doing well?" and "Is there anything you noticed I should have done differently?" Asking for specifics keeps your preceptor accountable and regular; meaningful feedback keeps you from being blindsided.

Stay in regular contact with your manager as well and ask for her feedback. If your preceptor or manager says you need to improve your time management, make sure you know what that means. "What would look differently when my time management has improved?" Ask for measurable goals. "Time management" is vague but "no overtime" is measurable. "Critical thinking" is broad, but "recognizes change in patient's condition" is specific.

Your preceptor is expected to complete either a paper or electronic orientation checklist on you. Typically, your orientation competency checklist needs to be completed before you can be taken off orientation. It's the preceptor's responsibility, but you can help by reminding them.

For example, if you just inserted a nasogastric tube (NGT) for the first time, prompt your preceptor to check you off on the skill. Being checked off means you are competent to perform the procedure.

What if you don't encounter an experience during orientation? You may not have had the opportunity to manage a patient on a PCA, for example. It may be 2 years down the road before you ever receive an order to use a blood warmer. If it's your first time using any device, or performing any procedure, you should be proctored. Print out and review the written procedure before you do it for the first time and ask your charge nurse to supervise you.

YOUR PART

In return there are things your preceptor will expect from you.

Be on time. Already mentioned, but it's worth emphasizing again.

Ask questions. Nurses are actually wary of new nurses who do not ask questions. Your preceptor is going to use acronyms you don't understand, and words that only make sense at your facility. Just ask.

Asking questions shows you are teachable and curious, both qualities of an inquiring mind and of a good nurse. No one is going to judge you for asking. Some nurses don't ask because they think their question is too basic, or they think it's something they should have learned in nursing school. Consequently, some nurses with several years of experience still don't know what bubbling in the water seal of a chest tube means for sure, but they are afraid to ask because they think they "should" know this by now. Don't be that nurse. You will find there are plenty of things you were not taught in school, such as management of temporary and permanent pacemakers, and ST depression on an EKG. Never stop learning and never stop asking.

Be open to constructive feedback. Above it was noted that it's the preceptor's job to give feedback and it's yours to receive it. Be open-minded and take to heart what is said. Know that a new nurse who seems unwilling to take constructive feedback is going to have a hard time succeeding. It's important to earn your preceptor's trust by accepting feedback.

TIME MANAGEMENT

Time management is one of the most common challenges for a newly licensed nurse. The secret to time management is prioritization. Prioritization and time management are two sides of the same coin. In fact, I would say time management is not possible without prioritization.

Here are some essential prioritization tips for you.

Prioritizing

Shifts rarely unfold in a pre-planned, linear fashion. Patients' conditions change in a heartbeat, and unanticipated admits show up at the same time as a rapid response is called on another patient. Meanwhile call lights are going off and you haven't gone to the bathroom, much less had lunch.

When confronted with multiple tasks and demands, how do you decide what to do first? Choosing to do one thing at any given point in time also means choosing not to do something else. You will always have competing demands and therefore it's imperative to prioritize your choices. Base your decisions on patient safety and time-sensitive activities. Be clear about the rationale for your decision and be able to speak to it.

When deciding what to do first after handoff report, ask yourself in what order you should see your patients. Use the criteria of safety, time-sensitivity, and scope.

- **Safety:** Is anything fatal? Is a patient unstable? Would a delay cause harm?
- **Time-Sensitivity:** If all your patients are stable, is there anyone going to surgery right away? If so, you have certain things to check before transport arrives. Is the consent signed and in the chart? Have valuables been checked if they are not returning to their room? Were a.m. meds given or held? Were a.m. labs checked?

- **Scope:** Which tasks can be delegated to a nursing assistant or patient care technician? "Alma, can you please grab some creamer for Patient A and take it in when you go to do his vitals? Thanks so much!"

Your preceptor will help you identify tasks that:

- Are the **most** essential, such as physical assessment
- **Need to be scheduled** or given on time, such as medication administration
- **Must be done within a longer time frame**, such as an every-shift dressing change
- Are **not** essential but **improve patient care**, such as a warm blanket

Example
Let's say Patient A just returned from surgery, Patient B's IV is infiltrated and puffy, and Patient C needs assistance to the bathroom.

Seeing your post-op patient right away is a priority because of the three patients, Patient A is the least stable. At the same time, an actively infiltrated IV needs attention.

- Turn off the IV infusion and tell Patient B you will be back soon to remove the IV. This is immediate, quick, and temporarily takes care of the problem (time-sensitive).
- Assess Patient A. This is your priority (safety).
- Call your nursing assistant and ask her to please ambulate Patient C to the bathroom (scope).

Always have a plan and prioritize continuously. Without prioritizing, you will get caught up in whatever is facing you.

Example

Say it's 0730 and you start rounding on your patients.

- Patient A needs creamer to go in their coffee, and their IV is leaking. You turn the IV off. You go to the supply room to get gauze and tape to discontinue the IV.
- Patient B's IV is beeping downstream occlusion. At a quick glance, everything looks fine and you push the alarm off.
- You go to the kitchen to get creamer and return to Patient A's room, realizing you forgot to grab the IV start kit from the supply room.
- Patient B's IV is again beeping downstream occlusion. You go in the room, turn the alarm off again and go to the supply room to get an IV start kit to restart Patient A's IV.

Example

Here's a better version.

- Patient A's IV is leaking; you turn it off. You know he is very likely to go home today, and he has no IV antibiotics due, so you plan to discontinue it. You will bring the creamer soon.
- Patient B's IV is beeping, and you know kinked IV tubing is often the culprit, so you pull down the covers, straighten the tubing, and tape the tubing to keep it straight.

Example

Q: As another example, let's say you have both a wound care dressing and an antibiotic due at 1400. Which will you do first and why?

A: Hang the antibiotic first because it's time-sensitive. A dressing change can be rescheduled without harm.

Procrastinating

Procrastinating is the opposite of prioritizing. It's avoiding doing things you may be uncomfortable doing, or things you dislike. Be careful you are not unconsciously gravitating to comfortable tasks as a way of avoiding new RN skills. Chatting with your patients or providing direct care when you are behind in passing your meds may be a function of your comfort zone. Generally, growth and learning take place when we're pushing ourselves and are uncomfortable.

Make a checklist to help with your time management. It may be a checklist for regular and expected tasks, such as:

0730 Patient assessments
0830 Start med pass
0930 Document assessments if not already done
1130 Fingersticks and correction scale insulins
1300 Review and update care plans

On night shift, add in assessing for sleeping pills early in case you need to call a doctor. Refer to your checklist during your shift to gauge if you're on time.

Documenting

Make every attempt to document in real time. You may think you don't have time, but it saves time in the long run. A sure way to guarantee being overwhelmed at the end of your shift is to put off documentation early in your shift.

Batching Tasks

Batching is the result of anticipating, and anticipating is a construct of critical thinking. Batching is bringing Patient A creamer, a two by two, and tape to discontinue the IV in one trip.

Batching and anticipating is grabbing a consent form and the NPO wall sign when you hear the doctor explaining the risks and benefits of the surgery your patient will have later in the day.

Anticipating and Planning

Have a "What's the worst that can happen?" mindset. Always anticipate what could go wrong and the worst that could go wrong, so you'll be prepared and you won't panic.

- When starting an IV, anticipate you may not get it at the first stick. By anticipating what might go wrong, you take two catheters into the room. This saves you a trip back to the supply room. What other supplies might you need?
- The monitor tech calls and tells you to immediately check on a patient because the leads are off. What's the worst that could happen? You could find the patient pulseless and unresponsive. Running down the hall, you rehearse what you'll do. Call a code, stay in the room, initiate basic life support. When you get there, your patient is talking on the phone. Thank goodness!! But you were ready to respond if the worst had happened.
- You survey the empty room where your patient will be returning from surgery. Make sure there is an emesis basin or bag in the room. Is the SCD pump in the room and ready? Is there a water pitcher in the room?

FIND YOUR HIDDEN RESOURCES

You'll notice that many nurses—the best nurses—just always seem to know who to call to get things done. And oftentimes, the people they call are not the ones with numbers listed on the back of your badge. It's Edna, the cheerful and efficient house-keeper who will help when you really need a room turned over fast. It's Erlinda, the dietary aide who will get a tray for your patient before the next scheduled meal time because he's been in Cath Lab all morning and hasn't eaten since yesterday. Get to know these key people who make things happen and learn their names and numbers.

Likewise, start your own phone list and add to it. Your floor's case manager, doctors who practice on your floor, and the best pharmacist to go to with questions. At the beginning of your shift, get the respiratory therapist's number and his name. Call for any respiratory-related question.

DELEGATING

Delegating is crucial to your success. Always help with patient care when you are able, but if you are regularly spending time turning, cleaning, and feeding and you are not completing your RN tasks on time, then your problem could be a failure to delegate. Your nursing assistant or patient care technician cannot respond to IV alarms, pass meds for you, or assess your patients, but he or she can assist your patient to the bathroom.

Delegating is hard for most newly licensed nurses because you want to help whenever there's a need. So if a patient says, "Can you get me some water?" you do. And when you return with the water, and they say, "Can you get me some more tis-sue?" out you go to the supply room. You want to help and get them what they need. But in the meantime, you haven't done any assessments or started your med pass, and another patient is waiting in agony for their pain medication. So you can't prioritize based on "who's in front of me now."

Partly it's about understanding your role. Think about it. If a doctor came in and started fetching water and taking patients to the bathroom, it would be very helpful. Or would it? If a patient was waiting in surgery or he was called to see a crashing patient in ICU, then fetching water and tissue begins to look less helpful. Most staff on the unit can fetch water. But only the doctor can perform surgery or give orders to stabilize a crashing patient.

Sometimes the nursing assistant can be older than you. Barriers to delegating include being reluctant to ask someone older than you to do something. The key is to be respectful and express gratitude.

Delegating Upwards
There's also upwards delegation.

Rapidly changing patient's condition is beyond the newly licensed nurses' ability to manage and you need to call for help, called delegating upwards.

Recognize your limitations and delegate upwards.

REFLECTIVE JOURNALING

As a newly licensed nurse, you will experience stress, compassion fatigue, and performance anxiety. Emotional pressure is common in nursing.

Feelings
Journaling can help you in many ways during orientation. Start a journal and write down the day's events. Reflect on what

happened. When you journal, write whatever comes to mind. Don't censor yourself. The journal is for you.

Be honest. You will gain more insight. This is a personal journal, so write what will be helpful to you for future reference. Don't identify people by name. Keep it personal, confidential, and private.

Emotions you experience during your shift need to be processed, but there is usually no time in the moment.

You will feel guilty, angry, fearful, sad, and the whole range of emotions. Do not act directly on strong feelings in the moment but do reflect on them. You need to examine your emotions. Get the negative feelings out by talking to someone you trust and exercising.

If the shift went poorly, if you were disappointed in your performance that day, reflect on exactly when things changed. What was happening? What could you have done differently if the day were repeated? Could you have asked for help before the tipping point?

Journaling Examples

Today I discharged my first patient. He personally thanked me for taking good care of him. I was surprised how good that felt. My preceptor said I was doing well, and I passed meds on 2 patients.

It was an awful day. A doctor asked me to get a simple oxygen mask and I grabbed a non-rebreather. I was supposed to get my patient with a chest tube up but I was too afraid. What if I disconnected it by mistake? But I did insert an ngt and it was insanely exciting to get drainage return.

Time goes by fast and soon, in month two or three, you will read your early first entries and be amazed at how far you've come. Give yourself credit for your progress.

CARING PRACTICES

Caring is really the core of nursing. Caring is preserving the dignity of patients at all times. It's never letting them know, for example, that the odor from their Stage 4 wound is turning your stomach. It's talking to your unconscious patient. It's praising a patient for passing gas after surgery. Caring and skills are intertwined. It's being competent and compassionate. We all committed to be caring, competent, and compassionate when we became nurses.

But there are times when that commitment is challenged.

DEVIANCY AND MORAL DISTRESS

One day on my Tele unit, I was assigned to care for an inmate who was there as an overflow patient because the correctional unit was full. There were two guards in the room and two seated outside the room in chairs. With his blond hair and smooth baby face, he did not look like a hardened criminal. Turns out he had committed an unthinkable act on a three-year-old little girl. All day long, I had to compartmentalize that information in order to care for him. Over and over, I would put the story, his crime, the little girl, all of it, into a little box, close the box, and put the box high up on a shelf, until he became just a person and a patient in front of me. A patient without context or background, just a patient who needed his IV re-started and his meds given by me, a dedicated professional.

I believe every human being is owed respect if only because life is sacred. Reminding yourself of your values helps change your perspective and focus when faced with moral distress.

Another time I was floated to the correctional unit. I watched a young man dying from AIDS and asked if his mother or family was going to be allowed to visit. The answer was no; it was against the rules for inmates to have visitors in the lockdown unit. Being a Mom myself, I found that very sad and distressful, but I had a job to do, which was to care for my assigned patients. As sad as I felt, what would help my patients the most in the moment was for me to be composed and competent.

When I first worked with inmates in the lockdown unit of our hospital, I would curiously ask the guard what were they in for, what was their crime? The guards always responded with "I don't know." I quickly learned that an admitting diagnosis of a fractured orbital was always caused by "falling off the bunk" and never "attacked by another inmate."

I learned not to ask, and then to cope. I learned not to wonder. Disengagement is a coping skill sometimes needed in nursing.

No matter what specialty you are in, there will be moral distress. Nurses in ED deal with patients seeking drugs and trauma victims. L&D nurses help moms deliver stillborn infants, or infants born addicted to drugs. ICU nurses care for unconscious patients on vents who should be allowed to die and have to deal with futility of care.

The key is to disengage but not to detach from your feelings. To compartmentalize as a coping mechanism, but to remain whole.

COMING OFF ORIENTATION

You've been checked off on everything, and it's time to come off orientation and practice on your own.

Some newly licensed nurses are eager to come off orientation, ready to assimilate all they've learned and put it into practice—their own nursing practice! Some are frankly tired of hearing yet another nurse say, "this is my way of doing it" and are impatient to finally start doing things their way. Others are terrified, and some are both eager and terrified.

What if you feel hesitant to be on your own, but your manager said it's time? If your preceptor, educator, and manager feel you are ready, chances are you are ready. They have enough experience to know. Trust the process. You are never alone. You are part of a team with a lot of resources. You have a nurse on either side of you, and a charge nurse. Be sure you've memorized her phone number and be sure to acknowledge how far you've come!

CHAPTER 3

SHIFT WORK AND WORK-LIFE BALANCE

It's a lifestyle adjustment to work in an industry that is 24/7, 365 days a year. As a nurse, your schedule is one of the most important factors in whether or not you are going to be happy with your job. I go so far as to say it's the most important satisfier. After all, your work schedule affects you, your friends, your family, and the whole of your life.

Expect to work half of all weekends in some form or another. You might work every other weekend or be required to work four weekend shifts per month. You may have self-scheduling or have a master rotating schedule, such as Monday, Tuesday, followed by Saturday, Sunday, Monday, Thursday and then repeat. Sometimes your schedule can be negotiated to meet your needs.

Michael did not like working weekends as his wife works weekends and it interfered with childcare arrangements.

He spoke with his manager, but she was unable to accommodate his request.

Lisa wanted off on Saturdays during football season to attend her son's games. She offered to work every Sunday as a trade-off. Lisa's manager agreed.

Often if you can present a solution to your manager or scheduler that meets the needs of the floor as well as your own needs, they'll agree. What Lisa did right was to acknowledge the needs of the unit and suggest a solution.

Once you are off of orientation, you can switch shifts with a co-worker. There are some great phone apps that make switching shifts with a coworker easy. Find out which app the nurses on your floor are using.

Switching has to be within the same role. So you can switch with a fellow bedside clinician, but not with a charge nurse. The charge nurse could work as a bedside clinician, but you can't work as a charge nurse.

Switching also cannot incur overtime. If your pay period is two weeks long, you can't ask a nurse to work the last Friday of the pay period in return for you working the first Monday of the next pay period. Since the trade is in different pay periods, it would put both of you into overtime.

WORKING NIGHT SHIFT: LOVE IT OR HATE IT

Most nurses will tell you they either love working night shift or they hate it.

Love It
There are some real advantages to working night shift. The really great thing about working nights is how much you will learn. You have time to think and process and not just to react.

You have time to read and digest doctors' progress notes, to process information, and to begin to connect the dots.

Some new nurses prefer night shift because of their coworkers. I've heard some of the younger nurses say they absolutely love working night shift because more of the younger nurses are on nights.

Night shift teams have a high level of camaraderie. They bond through the relative solitude. There's a lack of admin types. Surveyors typically never do site visits on nights and the majority of the hospital staff is home sleeping.

Another benefit is you probably won't need an alarm clock to wake up when you're working nights. You will wake up automatically. Being exhausted does help you fall asleep but staying asleep can be another matter.

There are downsides, of course. You may feel a little isolated or cut off from information. Some hospitals have educators who work night shift, but these are few and far between. Some managers make a practice of regularly checking in with their night shift, but not all do. To stay in the information loop, check your email and read flyers. Typically, you'll be given information at change of shift through huddle notes.

Hate It

I just can't do this. I'm tired all the time. No matter how hard I try, I just don't sleep well during the day. I wake up every two hours to go to the bathroom, and I just can't stay asleep. I get up around noon or one and that's it. It's not that I feel rested—it's that I can't sleep anymore. I'm like a zombie. Then if I have to go in that night, I face hours and hours ahead of me staying awake. It's exhausting.

When I get to work, I'm actually better the first night on, maybe it's adrenaline. The second night is tough because I know the patients and it's more monotonous. If I sit down between 0200 and 0400, I can hardly stay awake.

For nurses with depression or any other mental health conditions, working night shift can exacerbate their condition. It interferes with your metabolism and circadian rhythm. Speak to your manager about transferring to day shift and monitor yourself for early warning signs. See your provider if you experience any symptoms.

Sleeping

When on nights, many nurses prefer to work their shifts all in a row if possible, to avoid sleep disruption. Here's how one nurse plans her sleeping:

The night before my first scheduled shift, I stay up as late as possible. Usually until midnight or even 1:00 a.m. I go to bed and sleep as late as I can. Then I get up and eat, take a shower, and go back to bed to take a nap between 1400 and 1600. I go in to work at 1900. Then when I get off the next morning, I'm able to go right to sleep. I like to schedule my nights together and have at least two days off between my work stretches.

Another nurse said, "The hardest part is sleeping through the normal daytime noise that is just always going on. Kids are outside playing, your neighbor is mowing his lawn, dogs are barking."

Staying asleep long enough can be difficult. Your bladder is on day shift time and it'll wake you up. Try to get up briefly, go to the bathroom, and get right back to bed. Don't look at your phone. Don't engage as your mind will become more alert.

Regardless, try to sleep as long as you can. If necessary, put a note on the door saying "Day Sleeper, Do Not Disturb," so FedEx and UPS won't ring the doorbell.

If you are struggling to catch sleep as a new nurse on night shift, make it a priority to figure out solutions that work for you. Some nurses take melatonin before bed, some cut blue-light screen time back a couple of hours before sleep.

The most frequent sleeping aid I hear about and recommend is blackout curtains. They trick your body into thinking its nighttime. Think of the times you've slept in a hotel and slept in later than usual because the room is completely dark.

Another help is white noise. Having a low constant noise, like a fan, helps you tune out the intermittent loud noises outside your room. It can lull you to sleep and help you stay asleep.

Many nurses sleep until noon after their last shift on and then flip right back to their regular sleeping schedule on their days off. Give yourself enough time to adjust and find out what works for you.

Driving Home

A big caution on driving home. When you get off work and are driving home, be extra careful. Driving is a monotonous task and driving when you are sleep-deprived is a serious, known hazard.

Lower your windows, call someone and talk to them (hands-free, of course) all the way home. Don't let your car get toasty warm in cold weather if you have any distance to drive whatsoever.

The recommendations from the National Sleep Foundation (NSF) are even more strict. The NSF says that "if you find yourself turning the volume of the radio way up and opening the car window in an effort to combat sleepiness . . . you should immediately pull over. These tactics do not work effectively and are a serious warning signal that you are too fatigued to drive." Long blinks are a warning sign that you are about to fall asleep at the wheel.

The NSF further said, "Cognitive impairment after approximately 18 hours awake is similar to that of someone with a blood alcohol content (BAC) of 0.05 percent. Cognitive impairment after 24 hours awake is equivalent to a blood alcohol content (BAC) of 0.10 percent, which is higher than the legal limit in the U.S."

While you are at work, you are on alert and maintain a protective vigilance that helps keep you from making errors. But once you clock out, that protective vigilance fades.

Once while working nights I stopped to buy groceries. I went home and put them away, then went to bed. Later that day, when I got up, I couldn't find the carton of eggs. I was sure I had bought a dozen eggs. They weren't in the refrigerator. They weren't on the counter. I looked in the car. Maybe I just thought I bought them? Sighing, I opened the freezer to take something out for dinner, and guess what was there? A carton of eggs.

I had driven home fine and even gone shopping. But clearly, I was not in a state of vigilance. I was on dangerous auto-pilot.

Witching Hour

Some people will conversationally say, "Oh, yeah, I work nights, too." Then you ask where they work and they say, "I'm a waitress, sometimes I have to work till midnight. Once I didn't get off until 12:30!" There's no comparison between working late into the night and working through the night until the sun rises. Staying up late, getting up early, and never going to sleep at all are three different things.

We've all stayed up late until 0100 and 0200. Going to a party, maybe traveling, just being a night owl. Likewise, we've all gotten up early. I've gotten up at 0400 for a ski trip or to catch a flight. So I figure staying up late takes you to 0200ish. Getting up early starts at 0400ish.

But being awake at 0300 is neither staying up late nor getting up early. For me, it's a time when I'm not hard-wired to be awake and conscious. I call it the witching hour, and it's between 0200 to 0400.

My body knows this. Between the hours of 0200 and 0400, if forced to stay awake, I go into a mini-hibernation. It reminds me of times I've been outside in very cold weather and had mild hypothermia. My metabolism slows down and so does my brain. I get cold and can't really talk much. I used to laughingly tell my night coworkers ahead of time that at 0200, I would not be verbal.

The amazing thing was that right around 0430 to 0500 I would brighten up, be talkative, efficient and productive. Peeking out of a patient's window and seeing the black lighten and turn to gray and then glimpse the sun rising made me come alive again. No matter how sleep deprived I was, my body would wake up.

Napping and Breaks

Some nurses proclaim how long it's been since they ate or had a bathroom break almost in a bragging manner. Missing breaks and meals is not a badge of honor. Do your best to take regular breaks, and report to your charge nurse if you are unable to take a break. It is their job to provide relief so you can break.

When you are on a break where you are required to clock out, typically your lunch break, you are not working. Pass your phone to your break buddy and take a short nap. Set your watch to wake you up or have a coworker call you. Of course, follow your hospital policy, but know that being on a non-paid break means you are not available and are free of all duties.

Drink coffee during the first half of your shift but switch to water for the second half. Avoid energy drinks. Avoid high glycemic foods such as doughnuts because your blood sugar will rise, leaving you sleepy and feeling not only worse than before, but guilty. Bring portions of nuts, cubed cheese, or cut-up fruit to snack on.

If you feel yourself falling asleep, do a few lunges or take the stairs up or down a flight.

WORKING HOLIDAYS

Holidays can be tough for nurses.

Your first holiday season working as a nurse can hit hard. It's important to accept the inevitability of working holidays and choose to remain as positive as possible.

In most clinical jobs as a nurse, chances are good to excellent that you are going to work some holidays. Health care is 365 days a year, around the clock, and front line nurses are on duty.

In a hospital, different units may have different ways of scheduling holidays. Typically nurses have to work at least one and maybe two of the three major holidays—Thanksgiving, Christmas, and New Year's. Most hospitals try to have nurses work only half the holidays.

But without knowing the exact number, you definitely are going to work some holidays. Being new, seniority will likely play a role in who has to work which holidays.

Being away from family on holidays is actually a loss and can feel like grief. Some families will be very disappointed that you won't be there, and some may not be understanding. You may be asked, "Well, can't you just get off early in time for dinner?" or, "Have someone work half your shift so you can be with us." They don't know it just doesn't work that way.

Some nurses make other arrangements with their family to celebrate at a different hour or time. A holiday can be celebrated whenever you and your family decide.

Just like most things, there are two sides to the working-on-a-holiday coin. There are actually some benefits to working on a holiday. For one, there's usually holiday pay or premium pay. It's nice to have a plump paycheck around the holidays.

Holidays can be joyful, but holidays with family can also be stressful. For some nurses, having a reason to opt out of the holiday is actually a relief. If you're at work, you don't have to cook and clean up and you don't have to spend time with family members you don't love seeing.

The truth is, once you are at work, the outside world fades away and you are too busy to think much about what you're missing. Patients are all very sick because any patients who can possibly be discharged home are discharged home before the holiday. You soon see that some patients have no visitors and you are their primary human contact on that day. You have more time with your patients because overall it's quieter with no scheduled surgeries and no planned procedures.

There's camaraderie among the staff who work holidays. Often a potluck is organized. Doctors may round in Hawaiian shirts or equally casual dress. There is a nice chill vibe. Embrace your work family. You're all in it together.

MEAL PREPPING

Starting your first job as a nurse can throw you off of your routine. Being out of routine can set you up to make poor eating choices, such as relying solely on cafeteria food. Start with good habits that you can build on, and not poor choices that you have to reverse later.

Planning your meals is essential to staying healthy. Build meal prepping into your routine.

On your days off, shop and plan your meals for your next work week.

The right containers will help make your meal prepping successful. Buy containers that you can eat from and that go from refrigerator to microwave. Glass containers are better for the environment than disposable containers and Ziploc bags.

You will save money and calories by staying away from the cafeteria and you'll have choices that are right for you. You can start out by portioning out seasonal fruit for snacking in several small containers and soon you'll see how easy it is.

Try cooking some chicken breasts on your days off and slice it for salads and for whole wheat sandwiches another day. The Crock-Pot is your friend and the Instant Pot can be your best friend.

Having your own, planned food at work is important because otherwise your appetite is hostage to what's in front of you. It's easier to resist fresh, glazed doughnuts when you're not ravenous!

WORKING OVERTIME

Working overtime can be tempting but it's also a trap. In most facilities, once you get on the informal "yes" list, you will be called frequently. I've even seen managers put mild pressure on new grads who are eligible for overtime by personally appealing to them. They will say they are personally counting on you and your natural response is to please your new boss. Make no mistake, this is pressure, but the choice remains with you. No one can say "yes" but you, and no one will say "no" for you.

The extra money is tempting, especially after having been on a student budget, but keep an eye on your taxes as well. It is possible to make more money in the short run only to end up in a higher tax bracket and pay more taxes.

Be careful not to live beyond your means or base your lifestyle on overtime wages.

Be wise and start saving money regularly now for your retirement. When you get a raise, increase your savings. You won't miss money you don't see.

See what tax shelters and matching funds your employer offers and take full advantage of them.

Most seriously, working overtime puts you at risk for burnout. In fact, it's not a matter of if, but when.

WORK-LIFE BALANCE

You most likely have heard a lot about work-life balance. Many nurses are driven types and that can translate to a life driven by work. It's been said the younger generation is better at work-life balance than previous generations, so good for them!

Hobbies

Some nurses actually say they are not creative because they think that having an aptitude for sciences means they can't also be artistic or creative. That's simply not true. You are uniquely creative and multi-dimensional. There is a whole separate part of you aside from your work self that needs to be nurtured. Interests may have been put on hold during school, but it's time to pursue your passions. The single-minded, workaholic nurse must cultivate interests that feed her or him, such as gardening, hiking, dancing, crocheting.

You are establishing habits for a lifetime. If you don't establish habits to replenish yourself, you will dry up and have nothing to give.

It's also important to be authentic. Being authentic doesn't drain you, it keeps your tank full. It takes less energy to be you than to fake it and try to be someone you're not. If you don't know something, simply say, "I don't know," and if it's appropriate, "I'll find out." People respond to genuineness. Think how much you like people who are just themselves.

You have but to look around you to see nurses who have lost their compassion and even part of their humanity. Nurses who are jaded may be jaded due to responding to demanding patients and other conditions, but in the end, you—not your circumstances—are responsible for your own overall health.

PREVENT SICKNESS

Take care of yourself. It's common for new nurses to frequently be sick during their first year of work, but it doesn't have to be that way. Common self-care pitfalls of new nurses include:

- not getting enough sleep
- not eating well
- not protecting themselves against germs

Frequent exposure to new germs will definitely make you sick (and burn up your sick days). A few tips to protect yourself (as much as possible) from hospital germs include:

- following isolation precautions
- hand hygiene (number one!)
- cleaning high-touch areas and objects with a chlorhexidine wipe at work—your stethoscope, your ID badge, your pen, the keyboard you use. I even wipe down the surface of pumps and doorknobs.

Washing your hands and purposefully not touching your face with your hands prevents the most common mode of infectious transmission—contact. Train yourself to not touch your face.

CHAPTER 4

PRACTICE ENVIRONMENTS

UNHEALTHY PRACTICE ENVIRONMENTS

I really hope you do not land in an unhealthy practice environment your first year out. Unfortunately, it can happen. The bad news is that there is no shortage of unhealthy workplaces. If the situation is extreme, and your workplace is unsafe and toxic, it's especially hard for a newly licensed nurse, because then it becomes a matter of deciding whether or not you are going to honor your contract or commitment. That's a really tough spot to be in and one reason is you don't have a reference for what's acceptable and what's not acceptable. You may not know if the problem is you or if it's the job.

> I don't know what to do. I've been here for three months and I keep hoping it will get better. When I started, they promised me four weeks orientation, but on the third week said I had to be on my own because my preceptor didn't show. Last week a whole pack of twenty-five

oxycodone went missing somehow. My aide is usually outside smoking whenever I need them. I had to stay over last night because no one showed up to relieve me.

I have zero time to spend with my patients. My med pass takes two hours because I have the whole east hall, and I'm scared all the time. It's like I just pray I don't do anything wrong, because I might not even know. I'm racing at full speed to chart and draw labs.

I was doing some patient teaching on a discharge patient and they called to say I had to take report on an ED admit. I'm beginning to regret that I ever became a nurse. Did I waste four years of my life becoming a nurse?

There are indicators of unhealthy practice environments.

- **Constantly out of supplies.** You try to borrow from other units. Staff tend to hoard supplies and equipment. Some coworkers may seem to always have supplies, but you are out of the loop. You do not have the tools to do your job.
- **Aides are uncooperative to insubordinate.** Your aide never tells you when she is going on a break, and sometimes disappears altogether. Nurses are reluctant to ask the aides to do anything because of attitude.
- **Staff sleeping on the job when not on an off-the-clock break.**
- **Poor work organization.** You are never quite sure what your job is, there's poor communication and little support from supervisors.
- **High absenteeism.** The staffing office is scrambling for staff at all times. On duty staff are regularly asked to stay over, working 16 hour and longer shifts.

- **Desperation.** While you may have been desperate to get hired, you may not have noticed they were also desperate to hire you—or anyone. An example is offering a charge nurse position to a newly licensed nurse—it's a sign of desperation.
- **Extreme frustration.** Your own level of frustration is through the roof. Frustration is part of the job but so are satisfying and manageable moments. When you are frustrated from the beginning of the shift to the end, day in and day out, maybe it's the practice environment, not you.
- **Lack of dignity and respect.** Patients are treated disrespectfully or ignored.
- **Treatments or care are falsified.** In this situation, nurses are not able to complete all their scheduled care. So, for example, a dressing change gets charted as done, but doesn't actually get done. You change a dressing that smells, is heavy with drainage and clearly has not been changed recently but was documented as changed four hours ago.

Substandard Care

Disposable pads may cover soiled linen. Patients on bedrest are not turned. Vital signs may or may not be accurate. The staff feel forced to falsify information because the emphasis is on defensive charting and not on quality care. It stands to reason that it deeply impacts nurses who want to do the right thing but instead find themselves being dishonest, bit by bit. It causes moral distress. Staff no longer take pride in their care. Your license is at risk in this kind of environment.

Lack of Teamwork

In an unhealthy practice environment, everyone is in defensive and solitary mode. There are no approachable nurses because it's every man for themselves. Nurses won't make eye contact with you, for fear you will expect something from them. The teamwork is fractured, meaning it doesn't exist as a whole. Maybe two nursing assistants or PCTs work together, but you don't see them helping anyone else.

Policies Not Followed

Policies are not followed. You may be told about the policies and procedures, but you quickly realize that it's lip service only and they are not followed. In some cases, there are no policies and procedures to be found, or at least they are not visible and have no meaningful integration to practice. They are pulled out and dusted off for survey only.

As an example, you may be sternly told to never take a verbal order except in case of emergency or when it would break a sterile field, but your preceptor and other nurses do it regularly for a certain doctor. He rounds on the unit and says, "Start a tube feeding on Mrs. Alvarado" and next thing you see is the nurse entering it as a telephone/read back order.

This is essentially a broken organization where you are told one thing and expected to do something else, and it causes cognitive dissonance.

Example One:
Amanda was told that doctors have to explain the risks and benefits of a procedure or surgery before obtaining a consent, and she knows the doctor has not spoken with her patient about her procedure, but she is pressured to get the consent anyway. She questions and is told, "Oh, they'll get informed in pre-op. That's how we always do it. Get the signature, they're on their way to pick them up."

Example Two:

> *In the GI lab where I work, there is a tech whose job is to sterilize the scopes. On busy days, I've noticed that if a certain doctor is there in the endoscopy suite and wants to proceed with a colonoscopy, he will demand that he is provided with a scope whether or not the sterilization process is complete. He's extremely intimidating and demanding. So I've seen the tech shorten the sterilizing process in order to give him the scope he wants. But—gross! How is that okay?*

It's not okay. In both of these examples, staff begin to act as if it's not wrong, then as if it's normal, and finally as if it's expected. This is called normalization of deviance. For them it has become normal and a way to cope, so safety standards are eroded until everything is conditional and nothing is absolute.

Not Enough Experienced Nurses

You need to have experienced nurses on your unit that you can go to for support and consultation. When you work in a facility where the staff is unbalanced in terms of the ratio of newly licensed nurses to clinically seasoned nurses, it leaves you with fewer resources.

Unfortunately, in facilities experiencing high turnover, and on night shift, there may be a shortage of experienced nurses. Be sure and use your charge nurse as a resource.

Tough Culture

You should not be tested with the intent being to uncover what you do not know, but rather, you should be supported without judgment. In a tough culture, the support piece is lacking.

One form of tough nurse culture is "sink or swim." This is usually perpetuated by nurses who themselves were trained this way. They believe new nurses should be subjected to the same type of harsh orientation they experienced as new nurses. They may say things like "You nurses nowadays are coddled. We only had three weeks orientation and that was it. No one held my hand!" I've also heard nurses say, "Didn't they teach you that in orientation?" implying that you are at fault for not knowing something.

"Tough nurse cultures can develop in hospitals that are stressed by shortages and chronic high turnover" (Benner, 2009 p.267). It may be reminiscent of junior high or high school. Just remember that the behavior reflects on them, not you, and try to not take it personally.

Within a hospital, there are also subcultures, or mini-cultures within a culture. For example, the culture on day shift in L&D towards new nurses may be completely different than the night shift on L&D. Much of it has to do with informal leaders, management, and how long the staff has worked together.

Specialty Units

For whatever reason, specialty units such as ED and ICU can be breeding grounds for poor behavior. Specialty units attract strong personalities. Expertise is valued and incivility is excused as a tradeoff.

As a newly graduated nurse, know that if you work in an ICU or ED, chances are you will have to prove yourself. Nurses want to see that you're competent before they trust you to take care of "their" patients.

Here are some tips to help you succeed in the ICU:

- Befriend the Respiratory Therapist. He'll teach you everything you need to know about vents.
- Be humble. ICU nurses do not tolerate a know-it-all.

- Leave your patient fluffed and buffed. At the end of your shift, leave your room completely cleaned up and your patient spotless. Clean linen, fresh trach ties, oral hygiene, all complete. All lines labeled and dated.
- Don't leave IV solution bags empty or near empty. No one wants to start their shift by immediately replacing IV bags.
- Individualize your alarms—if your patient's current resting heart rate is 110, set your high alarm limit to 120.
- Jump in and help. If your coworker has a patient coming in from surgery, go over and jump in. You may not know how to hook up the lines, but you can position yourself across the bed, and help pull them over. You can take the Foley bag and hook it underneath the bed, and you can help turn them to get the sheets out from underneath. Initiative is highly valued, and your efforts will not go unnoticed.
- Likewise, when the phone at the desk rings, pick it up and say "ICU, this is Jamie, how can I help you?"
- When the printer runs out of paper, watch and learn how to restock it.

Queen Bee

A note on the Queen Bee. Toxic environments are populated by toxic people. Maybe you don't have a toxic environment per se, but you may have a dominant personality on your unit. A Queen Bee. The Queen Bee is easy to recognize.

A weak manager allows the strong Queen Bee to be her right hand.

The Queen Bee has referent power. That means she does not have legitimate authority like the nurse manager, but the nurse manager allows her to act like she's in charge. The tradeoff is that the manager has a strong nurse who is on her side and the Queen Bee has favoritism or special privileges with the manager.

The Queen Bee does not want to be a manager. She is not interested in developing budgets and disciplining staff and all of the other pressures and responsibilities. She does want to be acknowledged as having expertise and usually has seniority.

In many ways, once you give the Queen Bee what she wants, she is a great coworker. She is often knowledgeable and popular with staff and doctors. Just don't challenge her position.

For example, the Queen Bee may take pride in her guacamole dip. So as a new staff member, do not challenge her by bringing your even more delicious guacamole dip. She has established her domain.

Once in a consultant role, I was asked to educate the nurses on a Tele unit on pulling femoral sheaths. The nurses were required to attend, and it was instantly apparent whom the Queen Bee was. She was the one who rolled her eyes, sighed, and otherwise made it clear that I had nothing to teach her. Later we worked together as colleagues and got along fine, but only after I acknowledged her seniority and expertise.

Bullies

Ashley found herself nine months into ICU on night shift and was miserable. She dreaded coming to work in the evenings and was highly anxious and depressed. Ashley said the charge nurse gave her harder assignments than the other new grads. When Ashley asked for help from this particular charge nurse, she was neither helpful nor gave correct information.

What was my advice to Ashley?

I told her to first see her primary provider to get a diagnosis and treatment if needed. Anxiety is treatable. I also told her to access her employee assistance program (EAP) for counseling. Talking is extremely helpful. Then I advised her to start planning her exit so that by one year, when she is marketable, she can land a job in a healthier environment.

I also told her to start standing up to the bully, the charge nurse. For example, Ashley could ask her "When I asked you when Dr. Grimes wants us to mobilize his post-op open hearts, you told me they had to stay in bed for twelve hours. Was there some reason you said that when he prefers them up within four hours of surgery?"

Bullies always pick on someone vulnerable. It actually takes two to have a bullying situation—the bully and the victim. Once you stand up to a bully, they lose their power over you and quickly go to find someone else to bully. I learned this from personal experience when a doctor and a nurse bullied me.

In the case of the doctor who was a bully, I took him aside and said, "I know you want the best care for your patients. I do too. We have that in common. But you just undermined me in front of my staff. Next time something goes wrong, come talk to me in private and I'll follow up."

From that minute forward, he stopped bullying me and was always professional. We ended up with a mutually respectful, professional working relationship.

Another time involved a nurse colleague. She felt threatened by me and wanted to make me look bad in order to make herself look better. For a while, it was pure misery at work. I dreaded the days we had to work together. Then one day I found out she had undermined me to the charge nurse. I called her aside and said "Look. This stops now. We're colleagues and I'm done with your behavior." She stopped immediately and amazingly, we went on to work together successfully.

There are different variations of bullies. One is when older staff are condescending or scornful towards new staff. Sometimes bullying is very subtle.

A new grad named Lisa started in ICU. She was very conscientious and dedicated. One day she was caring for a forty-five-year-old female recovering from sepsis. Lisa was very empathetic and understood how uncomfortable the bristle of seven-day-old unshaven leg hairs is. She knew just how good it would feel to have smooth, shaved legs on the sheets. Lisa offered to shave her patient's legs and did so.

When she was done, the charge nurse came over said "Great, Lisa. Good job. So now everyone who follows you has to shave her legs, right? Way to go."

Lisa transferred out of the unit soon after and out of the hospital soon after that. A newly graduated nurse should never have been talked to in such a manner, but I wonder what would have happened if Lisa had replied "Are you saying I shouldn't shave my patients' legs?" or "That felt like a criticism. Is there something wrong with my patient care?"

TOXIC ENVIRONMENT

You may come to realize that the problem isn't you, but the work environment. Maybe there's a lack of support, or bullying, or some other kind of toxic environment. Unfortunately, some work environments are selectively toxic, meaning toxic to new nurses in particular. Toxic environments do not magically right themselves and become supportive, wonderful work environments. You will spend more time at work than at any other single daily activity during your life. It's just not worth it to be miserable when there are other options.

If it's your first job, don't judge all of nursing because of this experience. This does not represent nursing as a profession; it represents unchecked bad behavior and faulty management. When businesses are struggling just to survive, it's a jungle. It's not to say there are not toxic practice environments in larger, established, and financially stable organizations, but there are positive balancing aspects, if only more resources.

Once you realize you've landed in a toxic environment, the only thing to do is to strategically plan your exit. You cannot put your license at risk or risk harming a patient. Just be sure and carefully weigh the pros and cons because leaving during your first year or before the end of your contract has repercussions. *If you are able to stick it out, do so.*

If you are a newly licensed nurse and you have decided to leave, first get another job. It may be challenging if you are still in your first year, but it will be far more challenging if you are unemployed. When asked about your short tenure, simply say, "It wasn't a good fit. I look forward to working here where the mission and values match mine."

Employers do understand that sometimes nurses have to jump ship not because you are unreliable, but because some practice environments are untenable for anyone with integrity. Never say anything negative about a previous or current employer in a job interview. It will reflect more poorly on you than the employer.

HEALTHY PRACTICE ENVIRONMENT

Just as there are unhealthy and toxic practice environments, there are healthy practice environments. There is a Nurses Bill of Rights published by the American Nurses Society (ANA).

- Healthy practice environments have a zero-tolerance policy for abuse and disrespectful behavior in the workplace.
- There is meaningful recognition for the value each person brings to the organization.
- There is appropriate staffing.

Collaboration is essential in the workplace. Healthy work environments are linked to patient safety and improved patient outcomes. Unhealthy work environments are associated with increased conflict and stress among colleagues.

MANAGE YOURSELF

You cannot change other people, but you can change yourself. Being a better person makes you a better nurse.

- Do not indulge in gossip. Sometimes coworkers try to establish a relationship with you based on negative bonding. They will try to draw you into work drama. If a nurse is making unkind remarks about coworkers in the workplace, they will also make unkind remarks about you in your absence. Be aware of any cliques and avoid being drawn in.
- Become a skilled communicator. In fact, AACN said nurses need to be as skilled at communication as they are with their technical, clinical skills.
- Focus on finding positive solutions. As a nurse new to the unit, you have a fresh perspective.
- Act with personal integrity and hold others accountable to the same. Remaining silent is condoning the behavior. You are new but you have a right to speak up.

JUST CULTURE

One sure sign of a healthy work environment is one that embodies a just culture. A just culture is where you can report mistakes and near-misses without the threat of punitive action.

Nurse leaders have a great deal to do with the practice environment on their units. Your manager should have open communication with you and provide you with clear expectations. Your nurse manager should communicate frequently enough that you are not taken surprise by changes.

In healthy practice environments, nurses are involved in important changes and can give feedback. This may be through shared governance. There are opportunities for growth and your professional development is encouraged.

SUCCESS STORIES

If you are sinking, if you feel discouraged, don't give up.

Katrina was recruited from Canada and started in the ICU several years ago. She was bullied by the ICU nurses and has PTSD to this day from that experience. At one point she had her bags packed and almost moved back to Canada. Instead, she transferred to the ED where she is now an ED charge nurse, interim educator, and was nominated for Nurse Leader of the Year.

Don't give up and don't compare yourself to others. There are so many stories of nurses who had a rough start and now are successes and love their careers.

CHAPTER 5

DOCTORS

NURSES AND DOCTORS

Part of being a successful nurse is learning to work with doctors.

Nurses and doctors are trained differently, think differently, and are even socialized differently. It's not unusual to find some doctors who are socially awkward. Maybe it's because they spent years immersed in study and missed a lot of the normal socializing that takes place for most young adults.

By training, many doctors are loners and not team players. I've often thought nurses are trained to be team players and doctors are trained to be solo performers. Nurses are the volleyball players and doctors are the downhill skiers.

Nurses are detail-oriented and descriptive while doctors use fewer words and short, directive sentences. In a typical nurse-doctor interaction, by far the most words are used by the RN.

Nurses are often seen as more approachable than doctors, and that means patients will rely on you to translate what their doctor just said. The doctor will enter the room and deliver some information to the patient that typically is a one-way conversation, if a conversation at all. You will be needed to explain what was said.

Some doctors are more "old school" than others. On every unit there are doctors who bring in the most business and it's tacitly acknowledged that they have more pull. There may be a surgeon who wants things done his way and has his own specialized order sets.

On your unit, there will be a mix. In reality, doctor-nurse relationships range all the way from collegial to collaborative to adversarial. Doctors judge nurses based on their helpfulness, competence, and how well they communicate with them. Generally speaking, critical care nurses receive more respect from physicians than do nurses working on a med-surg floor.

For all of our differences, nurses and doctors both want the same thing—the best for our patients.

RESPECT IS EARNED

Respect from doctors has to be earned. You have to prove yourself in order to earn their trust. It can be frustrating when you feel a physician is not taking you seriously because you are new, but establishing your personal credibility takes several encounters.

Introduce yourself to every doctor on your unit. Extend your hand and make eye contact. This conveys respect for yourself, which in turn engenders respect from others. You want the doctor to have a visual image of you when you talk to her or him on the phone. It is harder to be rude when the person on the other end is not anonymous, but instead is a nurse they saw yesterday and will see again tomorrow morning. Take the first step and make yourself known.

HOW DOCTORS THINK

In order to team well together, we need to understand and respect our differences. Here's one example of how we think differently.

Nurses often think of time in terms of hours, but doctors also consider time in terms of twenty-four-hour units. Nurses are likely to look at hourly changes, such as an hourly change in urine output, while doctors will note the hourly amount and also look at the last twenty-four hours of intake and output. Both are important metrics, so it is helpful if you look at twenty-four-hour intake and outputs as well.

As an example of thinking in twenty-four-hour blocks of time, doctors will come in, evaluate the patient, order a drug or test or electrolyte replacement, and then order labs for the morning. The next day, twenty-four hours later, they look at the lab results to gauge the results of the interventions they ordered yesterday and to plan for the next twenty-four hours.

You will often hear providers say a patient is "headed in the right direction." Maybe your patient's white count today is 15,000. This is abnormal, but yesterday's white count was 22,000, so your patient with the white count of 15,000 is indeed "headed in the right direction." Always look for the trend and the context.

Read doctors' progress notes, consultations, and admission notes to gain insight into how doctors think. You will learn a great deal. Take advantage of doctors who are willing to explain and share information.

THE DOCTOR-NURSE GAME

There is a time-honored game to communicating with doctors. Stein first outlined the doctor-nurse game in 1967.

There are rules to the doctor-nurse game, which are based on deference and subordination of the nurse. The first rule is that there is no open disagreement. The second rule is that nurses' suggestions are indirect.

While much has changed decades later in the doctor-nurse game, versions of the game are still played. Still today, for your patients' sake, you need to learn how to approach a doctor with a request or proposal in a manner that promises the greatest likelihood of success. Nurses learn to become skilled at negotiating with doctors while avoiding engaging in a power struggle because that is never best for the patient.

Essentially nurses provide input and doctors make decisions based on that input, but it's all in how it's done. Instead of "Your patient needs two oxycodone 5-mg instead of one," you may hear a nurse say, "Your patient is on oxycodone 5-mg every four hours. She had a dose one hour ago and is still complaining of level seven pain. She said at home two pills work just fine," and wait expectantly.

It's okay to suggest an intervention that the doctor didn't include, but you feel is needed. If your patient is significantly short of breath and the doctor orders a CXR and O2 via nasal cannula, it's okay to also ask for ABGs.

CLINICAL KNOWLEDGE AND SCIENTIFIC KNOWLEDGE

As a nurse, you have clinical knowledge of your patient based on being familiar with your patient's usual responses. The doctor does not have the clinical knowledge that you do, but the doctor has more scientific knowledge.

For example, let's say you have a patient who's been on a dopamine drip for blood pressure and now it's down to a renal dose, which is not supposed to affect blood pressure. But with your patient, turning the dopamine down to a renal dose causes his blood pressure to bottom out. The doctor may disregard you, saying, "Dopamine at 2-mcg per minute does not affect the blood pressure" essentially trumping your clinical knowledge with his scientific knowledge.

By contrast, a wise, experienced physician will listen to an experienced nurse and give regard to her input. They realize that nurses are best positioned to identify subtle changes in condition and rely on us for this.

IMPORTANCE OF SUBTLE CHANGES IN CONDITION

Andrea's patient returned from Cath lab with a femoral sheath. Andrea pulled the sheath without complication, and held pressure on the site for twenty minutes until hemostasis was achieved. An uneventful sheath pull. The patient was instructed to lay in bed for three hours. The patient began complaining of back pain but had a history of chronic lower back pain. Andrea helped reposition him gently with a pillow propped on one side, which seemed to help. (It's okay to re-position a patient after a sheath pull, as long as you maintain extension and not flexion of the hip. Log-roll them). The next set of vital signs included a heart rate of 92.

So here were two subtle signs which only had significance when combined and in the context of just having had an angioplasty. Andrea suspected early signs of a retroperitoneal bleed, which is bleeding into the retroperitoneal space. There is no visible swelling or bleeding at the arterial insertion site. But there is back pain and an increase in heart rate.

Andrea called the doctor to report back pain and a heart rate elevated *from the patient's norm.* The doctor ordered an echo and sure enough, there was a bleed.

Don't disregard subtleties in condition. Pay attention to the small signs—such as a slight rise in heart rate. It could be early signs of sepsis, or a bleed, or some other serious condition. Patients usually give warning signs well ahead of time before they crash.

CALLING DOCTORS

The thought of calling a doctor on the phone can cause a lot of anxiety. During the first few weeks of orientation, it's customary for the preceptor to "carry the phone" and handle all of the provider communication. This shields you from encounters with doctors. During this time, watch and listen how your preceptor and other experienced nurses communicate with doctors.

Here's a tip—when calling a doctor, don't apologize. While it may be a social nicety to start with "I'm sorry to bother you" it also puts you in a subordinate position. There is no need to apologize. You've done nothing wrong by calling a provider about her/his patient when their condition has changed.

Before you place the call, ask if any of your colleagues also need to speak to the doctor, especially at night. This will be appreciated by the doctor, who would prefer one call rather than multiple calls from the same unit, maybe just after she or he fell asleep.

SBAR

Present your information in meaningful order using the SBAR model: situation, background, assessment, and recommendation. SBAR gives you a framework for organizing and sequencing information. SBAR is not rigid. You can and should modify it according to the situation. If you are calling a doctor who knows the patient, you may simply refer to the patient by name.

If you reach the doctor on call, you will have to give a brief pertinent history. Let's say your patient with a new onset GI bleed is on Coumadin or some other blood thinner. The primary doctor knows this but the doctor on call may not have this information. You can see where reaching the on-call doctor changes the conversation.

Have a Point and Get to the Point

Doctors are direct and purposeful in their communication. You must be as well. Don't include irrelevant information such as normal labs not pertinent to the situation. To learn how to be succinct, pretend that you are the doctor. You are out to dinner with your wife and children and receive a call about a patient you don't know. Now picture yourself giving pertinent information in a succinct manner, giving focused information, in order to help the doctor see the picture.

Let's say your patient is actively GI bleeding. You have the latest vital signs and the complete CBC from this morning.

The white count of 5,000 (normal) is not relevant. The hemoglobin (Hgb) of seven is relevant and significant to a GI bleed. Don't read information just because you have it. Think "What is the reason for reporting a normal white count in this case?" The answer is none.

Have a rationale for everything you do. What's relevant here are indicators of bleeding, the hemoglobin and hematocrit (H&H), and how the patient is tolerating the condition (vital signs and mentation).

Know What You Expect

Don't call a doctor without having an idea of what you need. When you are calling a doctor, typically you are expecting an order. The way you present the information is how you make your case for an expected clinical intervention. You must communicate in a manner that results in the best outcome for your patient.

For example, if you call to tell the doctor your patient is short of breath, has rales, and has pitting edema, what is it that your patient needs? What are you calling for? An order for a diuretic, for one. Maybe a chest X-Ray. If you get an order for Lasix 40-mg, IVP, fine. You expected that order and in fact gave specific information to get that order.

But if you don't know what it is you want, *you won't know if you don't get it.* So if the doctor orders a breathing treatment, you must compare their response with the expected response. A breathing treatment will not alleviate fluid on the lungs. Repeat your concern "The patient sounds very wet. Would you consider a diuretic?"

Clarify Orders

Once I was discharging a patient and took a final blood pressure on him while he was sitting in the wheelchair and dressed to go. The blood pressure was 178/92 and I called the doctor to see if it was still okay to go ahead and discharge.

He said "Yes, re-check blood pressure in fifteen minutes and if it's lower, send him home."

Ummmm ... Lower? How much lower? Fortunately, I asked him for parameters: "Can you give me systolic and diastolic parameters?" Now in this case, I knew the doctor was annoyed, and really just wanted the patient discharged. But I needed clear criteria for discharge in terms of blood pressure measurement. When I didn't get it, I asked for it.

"Discharge if the systolic is less than 150 and the diastolic less than 85." Perfect.

What I did was put the responsibility for discharge criteria where it belonged—with the doctor.

Along the same lines, sometimes you need to differentiate a conversation from an order. Conversations do not protect you; orders do. Ask, "Can you enter that as an order?" It should be crystal clear and include all relevant aspects of a proper order (frequency, duration, etc.).

When A Doctor Does Not Answer

There is hardly ever a time when you call a doctor and don't really need to talk with them. Therefore, it is not okay to not get a call back. Depending on the urgency of the situation, if a doctor does not return your call, call them back in fifteen minutes. Repeat again in fifteen minutes and then activate your chain-of-command.

So many times, I've heard nurses say, "The doctor did not call me back." That is not an excuse. The responsibility lies with you. I always ask, "And then what did you do?"

It would not be defensible for your patient to deteriorate because the doctor did not call you back. I have called the office or exchange many times and always ask, "And what is your name? Sheila, thank you, please have Dr. Ortho call me ASAP."

Fifteen minutes later: "Hi, Sheila! This is Beth" and so on. Hold Sheila accountable. Never neglect to get the name of the office worker or exchange.

Persist and document each and every time you call without a return call.

Taking Telephone Orders

Doctors should enter their own orders to avoid middle-man errors of transcription. Computerized physician order entry (CPOE) compliance varies greatly from facility to facility. There are cultures in some hospitals where nursing leadership looks the other way when the majority of orders are entered by nurses. I know of doctors who, when asked to enter their orders, go outside to their car, call the nurse, and say they don't have computer access. Some doctors just don't know how to do it. I think it takes far more energy for such work-arounds than to just learn CPOE.

> A newly graduated nurse named Raul called the doctor for his patient that was wheezing. The doctor responded with an order for albuterol and Raul said "Thank you! You'll be entering that order, right, Dr. Pulmonary?" . . . and the doctor did! This was a doctor who got other nurses in Raul's facility to enter his orders.

It is tough when your preceptor and the nurses around you enter orders for doctors, but do try Raul's method. Doctors are like anyone; they will get you to do things that are their responsibility—if you let them. It takes two to make a telephone order—a doctor and a nurse. There are doctors who enter their own orders in one facility and yet expect nurses to enter orders for them in another facility. This is because the facility allows it. And the bottom line is, what is safest for the patient? CPOE is safest for the patient.

ANTICIPATING ORDERS

It's important for you to anticipate orders.

Let's say you are on night shift and your patient has no morning labs ordered but some are indicated and it was clearly an oversight. Another example is, say you are on night shift, and your patient is having dialysis in the morning, call to ask what medications should be held if the doctor has not already given orders.

Or you may want a sleeping pill ordered just in case. If the patient has been unstable on every six-hour H&H but is now stable, chances are the doctor forgot to discontinue or change the frequency of the lab.

When you are on nights, it's even more important to look ahead and foresee what might be needed ahead of time. Call the doctor before 2200 rather than at 0100.

Talk to another nurse before you call and run your thinking/plan by them.

Case Study
Your patient has a drop in hemoglobin and hematocrit with no active signs of bleeding. Rather than immediately calling with an abnormal result, think it through. What are some possible causes of a decreased H&H? What orders and questions might you anticipate?

- Check their meds. You see that they're on Coumadin. Do you anticipate she/he will discontinue the Coumadin? Is Coumadin reversible? Is there a medication for that?
- What lab test might the doctor order to detect GI bleed?
- You would expect the doctor to discontinue the blood thinner, but what else would you anticipate?
- Recheck the H&H in the morning or at some point.
- Have they already been typed and screened? Crossmatch the patient for a possible blood transfusion.

- Will the doctor want a recent set of vitals? Have them ready and know if the current vital signs vary from the patient's baseline vital signs.

WHEN A DOCTOR SNAPS AT YOU

Sometimes a doctor will be irate and it has nothing to do with you. Let's say a lab is not resulted because of error. You could be back on your first day after five days off and it was night shift who is responsible for the error, but the doctor doesn't care who made the mistake. You are standing there, you have the patient now, and you are the target of their frustration.

It feels unfair but the best thing is to not take it personally and to do your best to fix it. "How about if we got the lab stat and I call you with the results?"

You can't control their response, but you can control yours. Remain professional and patient-centered.

GENDER

In the past, medicine has been male dominated, while nursing has been female dominated. This is changing, but it explains some old gender-based communication and behaviors between nurses and doctors. Male doctors may show dominance by impatience and interrupting.

Because of that history, you might expect female doctors to be especially kind and patient. This is not always the case. Ironically, some female doctors can be difficult when dealing with nurses. The reality is that many female doctors have the burden of fighting for respect in their specialties, especially male-dominated practice specialties.

DISILLUSIONMENT

There will come a time when you realize doctors are only human and don't always have an answer. Without consciously thinking about it, I used to believe that doctors would always have a solution. I remember when I realized that sometimes doctors are just trying different approaches and hoping for the best.

I was taking care of a post-op patient who had a carotid endarterectomy and his pressure kept increasing. I titrated pressors as ordered and kept calling the doctor after each failed intervention. I could tell he was increasingly impatient each time I called. Somehow I expected the doctor to have some magic answer up his sleeve to fix the situation, but he didn't. I was alone on the front lines to manage this patient and I remember the doctor actually saying "I don't know what else to do."

He wasn't being difficult. There are limits to medical interventions, and I learned to not take it personally.

CHAPTER 6

PRO TIPS FROM A–Z

This is a compilation of short tips in alphabetical order.

ASSESSMENT

Always pull down the sheets to assess a patient. By uncovering them, you discover things you would not otherwise see. For example, you may see a shortened leg in a patient with a hip replacement. The hip is dislocated. Look at the chest and abdomen for an implanted pacemaker, ACID, or implanted port. Patients may forget to mention these things. Scars may reveal old surgeries. You must turn the patient over to inspect their back and skin.

Learn to do a focused assessment. Assessments on the floor are much shorter than the assessments you performed in nursing school, because they are focused on the presenting problem.

ASSUMPTIONS

Your patient is a sixty-three-year-old male and his young, attractive daughter comes to visit. Or at least you think it's his daughter. It's his wife. Luckily you didn't say, "Hi, you must be his daughter. I'm Alesha, your dad's nurse today."

You will be surprised that some of your married patients have girlfriends or boyfriends. Girlfriends can show up to visit after the wife leaves, and vice versa. Never assume.

BACK CARE

You have only one back, and you must take good care of it. A good back is not only critical to your good health, it's your live-lihood. Do not lean over the side rail; take the time to lower the side rail. Raise the bed up to your height. Have your patients scoot over to the side of the bed you are on when starting an IV or doing a procedure. Use your knees to lift and learn the proper ergonomics to transfer and mobilize patients. If you are tall, you are more at risk for back injury over time because counter tops and other surface areas are not built to your height.

BLOOD CULTURES

Avoid drawing blood cultures from a central line as these samples are more likely to produce false-positive results. If a catheter related bloodstream infection (CRBSI) is suspected, the catheter may be used. Remove and discard the needleless connector in this case to reduce the chance of a false positive.

BLOOD TRANSFUSIONS

When transfusing blood, you know that the most serious reaction is an anaphylactic reaction. Anaphylactic reactions typically happen within minutes, if not seconds, of the donor blood coming in contact with the recipient's blood. So, stay in the room until the blood actually hits the vein, and then longer as your policy dictates. In other words, don't program the infusion pump and walk away.

Other blood reactions are typically not life-threatening. Know that it is common for a patient's temperature to elevate slightly during a transfusion—called a (non-hemolytic) febrile reaction. This is the result of the patient's antibodies attacking transfused WBCs. The donor's blood will never perfectly match the recipient's blood as there are thousands of known antigens. Patients receiving multiple units of blood may prophylactically be given an anti-pyretic. The point is that a slight elevation in temperature is an expected reaction to foreign antigens and does not constitute a life-threatening reaction.

Blood Screening and Type and Cross
A type and screen should be ordered if there is potential for a transfusion, but a transfusion is not likely. A type and cross should be ordered when the likelihood of transfusion is high. The advantage of cross-matched blood is that it's quickly available if needed.

When ordering a type and cross, the provider will specify how many units. The cross-matched units are then put aside and held for that patient. Typically, cross-matched blood is good for three days.

Practice-Based Evidence Tip
(See Chapter 9, Myths of Nursing Practice, for the difference between evidence-based practice and practice-based evidence.) When checking the H&H after a transfusion, I generally wait one hour if possible. Why? I have learned that if you check the H&H after, say fifteen minutes, the results will be lower

than if you wait one hour. Blood transfusion guidelines are to restrict transfusions to patients with less than a seven or eight hemoglobin. It could be that if you wait, your patient may not need an additional unit.

Generally speaking, one unit of packed red blood cells increases the hemoglobin (Hb) concentration by 1 g/dL in an adult, although it varies according to weight and blood volume.

Likewise, when a patient is actively GI bleeding you will get an H&H. Let's say the patient's Hb is nine. Chances are if you check it again in one hour, even in the absence of any further bleeding, it will be down. Just an interesting factoid noticed by me in practice (practice-based evidence). There seems to be a lag time when it comes to H&Hs.

BOWEL OBSTRUCTION

Many nurses don't know that there are bowel sounds with a bowel obstruction. They think that in the case of a bowel obstruction, all bowel sounds are absent. Not so.

Bowel obstructions can be mechanical, as in severe constipation, or paralytic, as in an ileus.

When you hear high-pitched, tinkling bowel sounds, especially in the upper quadrants, combined with abdominal distention, you most likely have an early partial obstruction. Anticipate a nasogastric tube to decompress the stomach. Patients with prior abdominal surgeries may have adhesions which can contribute to bowel obstructions.

CHAIN OF COMMAND

I jokingly tell nurses that activating the chain of command means passing your problem up the chain to the next person who makes more money than you.

The first person up the chain of command is your charge nurse, then your nurse manager. On night shift it's the charge nurse, then the house supervisor. They are there to help you and serve as a resource.

For example, if a doctor requests a supply, say a chest tube, that is not stocked on your floor, and materials management is closed, the house supervisor can get it for you. Likewise, if you have an angry family or patient, the charge nurse or nurse manager can come in and de-escalate the situation.

So don't hesitate to activate the chain of command. Your job is to provide patient care. You do not have to manage and take care of everything yourself. It's a team, and you are never alone.

CHEST TUBES

The main confusion around chest tubes is usually around the water seal and the suction.

Water Seal

The water seal chamber, which is connected to the collection chamber, acts as a one-way valve. Nurses often ask if bubbling in the water seal is a good thing or a bad thing. Well, the answer is, it depends.

If your patient has a pneumothorax (air accumulating in the pleural space), bubbling in the water seal is an expected finding. In the case of a pneumothorax, the purpose of the treatment is to drain the air out so the lung can re-expand. The drained air travels through the collection chamber into the water seal and creates bubbles. In this case, it's expected and therapeutic. Over time, the lung will seal itself off, the air in the pleural space will decrease, the lung will expand fully, and we've done our job.

But what about the patient with a hemothorax (blood in the pleural space)? In this case blood is being drained out of the pleural space. You see the blood accumulate in the collection chambers. But there shouldn't be air bubbles in the water seal because the patient does not have a pneumothorax.

In this case, the air is an unexpected finding for the patient's condition. The bubbles indicate there is an air leak somewhere in the system. Check the connections (where it's taped). The air could also be coming from the insertion site if the trocar has shifted a bit and is drawing in some air through the eyes of the tube. Clamp the chest tube as close as possible to the proximal end, nearest the patient. If the bubbling stops, the leak is at the insertion site.

If the bubbling doesn't stop, clamp the chest tube distal to the connection between the trocar and the chest tube drainage system tubing. The trocar is connected to the chest tube drainage with a graduated connector and taped over with microfoam surgical tape. If the bubbling stops, the leak is at the connection site. Remove the old tape, tighten the connection, and re-tape securely. Don't just tape over the connection and old tape.

Fluctuation in the water seal chamber is called tidaling and is a normal reflection of changes in intrathoracic pressure.

Dry Suction Control
Now let's talk suction.

The doctor will order a level of suction, say -20cmH20, which is a default setting and can be changed by simply adjusting the rotary dry suction control dial. The doctor orders the amount of suction, but the nurse makes the change on the device. In addition, there is a suction monitor bellows—resembling an accordion—that extends to a marker when the ordered suction level is achieved. Every time you enter the room, glance at the suction monitor bellows to confirm correct suction operation. Make sure the bellows is expanded across the suction monitor window to the marker.

The wall suction regulator should be turned to whatever is needed to cause the bellows to expand to the marker. It may be 120mmHg or higher. If the bellows are not expanded enough, increase the suction on the wall regulator. How much? However much it takes. The wall suction regulator does not confirm the amount of suction, the expanded bellows does.

Gravity

Remember that gravity is a force at play even when suction is removed. In my classes, I remind nurses of this basic fact. I jokingly tell them that if they don't believe this, just strip naked every five years or so, look in the mirror, and proof of the force of gravity will be evident.

It's better to mobilize a patient than to keep them on bedrest only because you do not want to temporarily discontinue the suction.

So accordingly, take your patient off of the wall suction and ambulate them unless contraindicated. Gravity is still at work, and drainage will occur. You do not need an order to take them off suction, and mobilization is highly important and beneficial. Doctors know they will be taken off suction when going for their daily chest X-ray to view the progress of their expanding lung.

When you first stand a patient with a hemothorax or pleural effusion up, there may be a gush of drainage. Likewise, when a patient with an abdominal surgical incision first stands up, blood or serosanguineous fluid tends to gush out of the incision site. This is not cause for alarm—the locus of gravity shifted when they went from supine to standing up, and the fluid that collected in that space can now drain out.

CHARTING

Keep on top of your charting. One thing is predictable and it's that your day is unpredictable! You may think you'll have time to catch up on charting later in your shift, but don't invoke the gods. You will get an unexpected admit or your patient will crash, and then you'll really be behind.

C. DIFFICILE (C. DIFF)

With C. diff, infection prevention and nurse leaders go into high action to prevent transmission and an outbreak. What's often forgotten is handwashing in patients. Encourage your patients to wash their hands before meals. Often when patients are in bed and their tray comes, they eat without washing.

If you recall, the mode of transmission for C. diff is fecal–oral. Bed rails and over-bed tables are high-touch areas, so keep them wiped down with a bleach wipe. If a patient's hands simply come in contact with a high-touch area that harbors C. diff, and then that patient touches their mouth, or eats, that patient may contract C. diff.

If there is an outbreak of C. diff, you will probably be using bleach germicidal wipes on your whole unit. Be very careful because just grazing your scrubs with a bleach wipe will leave unsightly bleach spots that do not wash out.

CODES

If your patient arrests, stay in the room or go to their room immediately. Do not leave. One of the worst things the primary nurse can do is to disappear.

When the rapid response team (RRT) and provider respond, they will ask for you. They will ask you what happened and why the patient was admitted.

Before you are ACLS certified, you will not know what to do in a code. One suggestion is to be the recorder if your facility permits. There is a clipboard with a code record on the crash cart, and the recorder is responsible for completing the form. It will have spaces to document what drugs were given, shocks administered, rhythm, etc. Take a look at the form next time you go to work.

The most important thing is to record time accurately. Do this by using one timepiece. It doesn't matter if you use your watch, or the clock on the wall, but just use the same one throughout the code.

You can see the problem if you document shock given at 1400 by your watch and CPR resumed at 1405 by the wall clock versus shock given at 1400 and CPR resumed at 1401 both by your watch.

The benefit of being a recorder is that it gives you a key role, so you can be useful and you can learn without undue pressure. With the clipboard in your hand, you will not be asked to push meds or grab a piece of equipment you are unfamiliar with. You gain exposure to codes.

Again, check with your facility if this is okay. Some facilities limit recording in a code to charge nurses only because the code forms were found to be incomplete when reviewed. Most call forms require the provider's signature, so be sure and get that before the ED doc goes back to the ED or the provider leaves.

Another role you can perform in a code is to perform CPR. Take the opportunity, you will not regret it. When performing CPR in real life, you may feel ribs crack and crunch below your hands. It feels awful, but don't break your stride and just keep going. If you are doing CPR, the patient is at risk of losing their life and cracked ribs are better than dying.

While the crash cart is open, take the time to learn which supplies are in which drawers. Picture yourself being asked to grab a twenty gauge needle. You will want to know where to quickly locate it.

CONFLICT

Once a nursing assistant I'll never forget named Annabelle called me aside. "Beth, when you start IVs you leave the bed a mess." I was shocked, my mind searching for my transgressions. Did I do that? Not clean up after myself? As it turned out, apparently, I would leave a spot (or more) of blood on the bed sheets or draw sheet, causing her to have to change the bed. From then on, I always placed a disposable pad underneath the patient's arm. Without intending to, I had been guilty of leaving the beds a mess. I realized that she took great pride in her work and always left her patients in tiptop condition, including the linen. Me leaving blood in the bed caused her extra work.

She taught me a lot that day. If you have a conflict with a coworker, take them aside, explain the concern and ask for what you want. Channel your frustration in the right direction, instead of bad mouthing them to other coworkers. Whenever I teach a class on professionalism, I think of Annabelle.

DEATH, WHAT TO DO
WHEN YOUR PATIENT DIES

When your patient dies, you may be the first line of comfort for the family.

Ask if you can give a hug if it is appropriate. You can provide tissues or get extra chairs for the family to sit in. You can say "I can't imagine what you must be going through."

Give the family some quiet time together.

There will come a time when either you must exit the room or you have to encourage the family to say their goodbyes and exit the room in order to free up the bed. This doesn't happen often, thankfully, but if the family has been there for an extended amount of time, it may be necessary to move the body to the morgue. This decision is up to the charge nurse, but here's a great tip when you need to leave the room and the family member is still very emotive or crying.

You can say "I know he was a teacher at West High. What subjects did he teach?" This immediately takes the listener or family member from the emotive side of their brain to the cognitive. They will stop crying and respond "He loved those kids. He especially loved teaching algebra."

We operate primarily from one side of the brain or the other at a time, either the cognitive or the emotive, and you don't want to leave someone in an emotional state. Now that they are in a cognitive state, you can ask "What arrangements have you made? Can I call Hillhouse Funeral home for you or get the number?"

EMOTIONS, MANAGING

A key part of being a nurse is being compassionate, but we have to manage our emotions.

Some nurses are easy criers. They tear up easily because they're empathetic. It's not that they want to—no one likes to feel out of control.

When you feel the tears threatening, try this trick. Perform a math problem in your head.

Do a multiplication table or add 6 + 17 + 2. This takes you from the emotive to the cognitive and dries the tears.

FEMORAL SHEATHS

For those of you who will be pulling sheaths, have the patient empty their bladder beforehand. A full bladder during a sheath pull can cause a vagal response. A vagal response is when the heart rate slows down, causing the blood pressure to drop. A sheath pull takes about a half hour, and it can take much longer if it takes a long time to achieve hemostasis. So be sure and start with an empty bladder. Keep in mind that patients who are obese, and especially those with a pannus, tend to bleed longer.

Never obscure the puncture site. Apply pressure proximal to the site and leave the site clearly visible. If you have ever observed someone pushing both hands flat down with a wad of 4x4" sponges, they have lost control. Best technique is focused pressure directly on the artery.

After hemostasis, check on your patient regularly by pulling the sheets down and exposing both groins. Compare the two and assess the puncture site. You may not recognize mild puffiness unless you compare it to the other side. The puffiness is swelling, or the beginning of a hematoma. Apply pressure and it will usually be reabsorbed.

Also check the pedal pulses bilaterally. Nurses sometimes become overly fixated on the pedal pulse to the point of ignoring hematomas and other much more common complications. During a sheath pull it is normal to obliterate the pedal pulse because you are compressing the artery that feeds it. It will return once you relieve pressure.

FOLEYS

Sometimes the urethra is difficult to visualize on female patients. If you tried for the urethra but instead catheterized the vagina, leave the catheter in place. Get a new catheter and try again. With the vagina now obstructed, you will be successful.

Always wait for urine flow before inflating the balloon. You can cause damage by inflating the balloon when it's not in the bladder. If you think you got in but aren't sure, do not inflate the balloon. Secure the tube on the thigh with a securement device or tape and wait. You usually get immediate urine return when it's in the bladder, but not always. I have waited several minutes in some cases, and one time, over twenty minutes.

Sometimes patients will say they "can't go" when they have an indwelling catheter. Just telling them to "go ahead and go" usually takes care of it.

After a Foley is discontinued, some patients have a hard time voiding. Morphine and other narcotics can cause this as well. The patient has the urge to go but isn't able. Give it some time, reassure them they will be able to go, run the tap water in the sink, and measure when they do go.

Keep an eye on patients who urinate small amounts. They can easily have residual urine from not emptying completely. This happens most often after surgery and the nursing assistant will typically not realize that the small amounts are not a good sign, they're an indicator of a problem. You must oversee the intake and output (I&O) yourself. Check with a bladder scanner if you have a concern.

> I was doing morning rounds and rounded on Edna, who'd had surgery the day before. I asked how she felt, and she looked uncomfortable and pointed to her abdomen. I pulled back the sheets and saw her abdomen was distended, and her bladder area in particular was sensitive to palpation. I immediately suspected residual urine and straight cathed her. She had 1800 cc urine return.

It was frustrating to know that she'd been uncomfortable and no one had recognized the problem. I looked at the I&O and saw what I expected to see—small amounts of 100ccs, 50ccs, maybe 150ccs. The night nurse did not recognize that these amounts are too low for a patient with a maintenance IV running at 150 cc/hr.

On the other hand, immediate post-op patients are usually dehydrated, and their urine output can be low for a few hours. Consider all the reasons for a low urine output and then differentiate the causes.

INSULINS

Basal insulins cover metabolic function in the absence of a normally functioning pancreas.

Therefore, they are not always held when a patient is NPO because the coverage is not for food, it is for metabolic activity. Check with the doctor before automatically holding long-acting insulin, especially glargines, which do not peak.

Long-Acting
Examples include glargine (brand names Lantus, Basaglar) and detemir (brand name Levemir). They start working within two to four hours. There is no peak. They are given once a day or twice a day.

Intermediate-Acting
NPH (brand name Humulin N) insulins are commonly prescribed insulins. They are prescribed once a day or twice a day. Nursing consideration: NPH peaks in six to eight hours, so around 1400 or 0200 be aware your patient can have signs of hypoglycemia.

Short-Acting
Short-acting insulins start working within thirty minutes to one hour of administration. Short-acting insulins should be

administered thirty to forty minutes before meals. Examples are regular insulin (brand names Humulin R, Novolin R).

Rapid-Acting

Rapid-acting insulins start working within fifteen minutes of administration. Nursing consideration: give within fifteen minutes of patient taking their first bite of food. Examples are lispro, aspart (brand names Humalog, Novolog).

IVs

Ask any experienced nurse and they will tell you that they have good days and bad days when it comes to starting IVs. Even when you have plenty of experience, there are the days when you can start an IV blindfolded and other days when you can't hit the side of a barn.

Take two IVs in the room with you when you go to start an IV. Don't waste time or test your luck by taking in only one IV, causing you to make two trips when you don't get in on the first try.

When starting an IV on an elderly patient with fragile skin, don't use a tourniquet. The veins are typically clearly visible and it's easy to stretch the skin to pop in your IV. Your IV is much less likely to "blow" in this case. Fragile veins cannot tolerate the pressure from a tourniquet and the pressure from the tourniquet itself causes it to blow.

A modified version of this is to apply a B/P cuff and inflate slightly and gently. It is less pressure than a tourniquet.

You'll hear the phrase "floating in an IV." Floating is gently flushing as you simultaneously advance the catheter. It can be very helpful in getting past valves.

From a nurse:

My ER RN mom taught me what to do if you have a pt (patient) whose veins always blow when advancing a catheter! Once you see flash, stay still & count to 5, then advance the slightest bit forward & introduce catheter. Veins can spasm when you put a needle into them. Counting to 5 lets them chill.

Using a vein finder is helpful for finding veins but is more helpful for locating and avoiding valves. Once you identify a valve, adjust your entry point above or below enough that your catheter is well clear of the valve.

Just because you got blood return and your IV looks good, doesn't mean you can't still have a slow infiltration. Your patient will complain of pain to the site and that's often a sign all is not well. Once a newly placed IV is in, patients don't generally complain of pain.

After two attempts, ask another nurse to start an IV on your patient. Know who to ask. Don't automatically ask an ICU nurse to come start your IV. ICU nurses typically have less experience starting IVs than floor nurses because so many of their patients have central lines. ED nurses have lots of experience but will often go for the antecubital and aren't available to leave the unit anyway. Nurses who work in procedural areas are usually highly skilled at placing IVs. Learn who the nurses are on your unit that are skilled at starting IVs.

When it comes to checking patency on central lines, remember there are two checks. You should be able to easily flush (1) and briskly aspirate 3 ccs of blood (2). You may find that you can easily flush, but that aspiration is sluggish. This is a sign of a partial obstruction caused by fibrin threads at the end of the catheter. It can be cleared by using a thrombolytic drug such as alteplase and save the expense of inserting a new line. Notify your charge nurse to find out your facility's protocol for using alteplase.

Continuous IV tubing is changed every ninety-six hours. and intermittent tubing is changed every twenty-four hours. Intermittent tubing is tubing which has been disconnected from the system, such as secondary tubing used for antibiotics. Leave the secondary tubing plugged in whenever possible to avoid multiple tubing changes. You can use the same secondary tubing for different antibiotics as long as they're compatible. Just have your preceptor show you how to backflush or back prime. By not breaking the system, you are reducing infection.

MANIPULATIVE PATIENTS

We don't always like the patients we take care of. The truth is, we don't have to like them. We have to provide the best care we can while being professional and maintaining a level of compassion. Some patients will test your nerves and your capacity to empathize. These are patients who appear to have limitless needs.

Some patients are rude, some are ungrateful, some are manipulative. Manipulative patients use coercive behavior to get you to do something. It's not always a matter of giving them what they want—with some people, the more they get, the more they want. They are never satisfied and you can't change that. Alternative suggestions offered are typically rejected.

We are taught in nursing school to understand that people who are ill experience loss of control and stress, which brings out their worst side. But I'm talking here about the person who is a manipulative person pretty much all the time and, of course, still manipulative when they're hospitalized. It's one thing to understand where their behaviors are coming from, but you are not expected to accept abuse.

The manipulative patient will somehow have you running all over the place with their multiple demands. You know you are being manipulated when you feel angry or irritated or have a feeling of having been hijacked. Trust your feelings. It's important to set boundaries with a manipulative patient.

Documentation

"Difficult patients who are more likely to sue are typically uncooperative, immature, dependent, and hostile." (Westrick, S. J., 2013, p 26).

It's even more important with difficult patients to provide consistent professional care. You are not expected to allow the patient to insult you, and limits on inappropriate behavior must be set. In your documentation, avoid labeling patients. Document their behavior, their concerns, and how you responded. Your documentation should reflect that you followed policy and procedure and acted as a patient advocate.

Set Boundaries

Never underestimate the skill of a manipulative patient. Your tools are recognition and setting boundaries. Recognize flattery as a form of manipulation: "I'm so glad you're here. That nurse last night was always late with my pain meds."

This is splitting behavior. Unless you believe there was a legitimate patient concern to follow up on, don't ask questions. Some patients manipulate through flattery and also through flirting.

People and patients who are manipulative know how to push other people's buttons with uncanny aim. If you feel a disproportionate rise in feelings, it's a sign that you are being manipulated.

Set appropriate boundaries early on. For example, if one nurse allows a patient in the kitchen, or brings in four extra chairs taken from other patient rooms, it will make it harder for every nurse following. Here are some tips.

- "That is not an appropriate thing for you to say here."
- "You cannot talk to me like that."
- Be helpful but don't be a doormat. "What else can I do for you while I'm here? I'll be back in an hour for hourly rounding."
- Stay calm. The behavior is not because of you.
- Maintain eye contact and use their name.

Some male patients will expose themselves and it's best to either not react or to firmly say, "You need to cover yourself." They are looking to make you uncomfortable, and if they get no reaction, they have no reason to continue.

"Joan" with Crohn's disease

As a student nurse, I once had a patient with end-stage Crohn's disease. She had a large, vertical, poorly-healing incision the entire length of her abdomen that was not approximated. It was infected and draining. It was held together by Montgomery straps laced across her entire abdomen in a failed attempt to hold the wound edges together.

The infected, draining wound was in contrast to her impeccably made-up face, styled hair, and beautifully manicured pink nails. She wore a burgundy satin dressing gown from home. On her bedside table she had stacks of documents and a BlackBerry. She looked like a businesswoman.

Her over-bed table held her hand lotion, a glass of orange juice, a water glass, and a phone. She was otherwise able-bodied and alert. She asked for a sip of orange juice and I gave it to her, holding the glass. The next thing I remember was being horrified as the orange liquid oozed out from her abdominal incision.

The other thing I remember is that, over and over, she had me move the objects on her over-bed table. I set the orange juice down and she had me move it one inch over. Then I fetched her lipstick and set it next to the hairbrush but that, too, was not right, and I had to put it on the right hand side of her phone.

When I finally was able to leave the room, I felt like a puppet on a string. I did not have the skills at the time to set boundaries with her, so I dreaded going in the room because I had no control over how long I would be in there.

I once talked with a nurse on her day off who was so frustrated with one patient that she talked non-stop for over twenty minutes. She had been assigned this patient two nights in a row and her coping skills were exhausted. The patient was insulting and had even told her that "my insurance pays for you and I expect good treatment." She remained professional but felt belittled and asked her charge nurse to change her assignment on her next shift.

This is to say that it's okay to ask for a change in assignment. Sometimes it's the best solution for extremely difficult patients.

"Kyle" the Drug User

Another difficult patient was Kyle. He was in his 30s and recovering from an abscess on his arm that required surgery and a wound vac. He was charming and sociable. He was also a drug addict. He did everything he could to get us to bring his Dilaudid before it was due, or to call the doctor to increase his dose. He stood in the hallway so we couldn't avoid him, while playing on his phone and complaining of a pain of ten.

I was assigned to him that day and dreaded every two-hour haranguing. I did not like the feeling that I was enabling his addiction. Then I realized that he was acting that way because he was an addict. That's what addicts do. Why would I expect differently?

Once I changed my expectations, I went up to him fifteen minutes before his next dose was due. "Kyle, how's your pain? Do you need your Dilaudid?" In this way, I took control. Once I didn't participate, there was no longer a power struggle.

How to Get Out of a Patient's Room

I consider politely getting out of the room of an overly-talkative patient a core competency. Getting out of the room while politely meeting your patient's needs is an acquired skill. "I would love to hear more, and I hope I can later. Right now, I have to see my other patients."

If you have a hard time getting out of your patients' rooms due to lengthy conversations, you will get behind. Don't allow yourself to be unwittingly hijacked. You must recognize when this is happening and learn the skill of tactfully extricating yourself. Watch what your preceptor does or says to exit the room while still meeting the patient's needs.

Always tell a patient when you will return and keep your promise. Remember to under-promise and over-deliver.

When going into a room where you anticipate you may have difficulty exiting, pre-arrange to have your preceptor or coworker call you after ten minutes. When your phone rings, excuse yourself to take the call.

Here's how one anonymous nurse describes herself when handling difficult patients:

I seem to do well with some types of patients. I pick up on the patient needs/wants, and while the first shift may be a challenge, subsequent shifts are usually better. I try to remember patient likes/dislikes/preferences (juice, ice, blankets, etc.). Before going into the room, I take a look at the available PRN meds (or what time next ones are due). Usually a lot gets "fixed" the first night. So, whatever is needed is ready for subsequent nights.

I remember not too long ago I had the "drug seeker" type in bed A. If there's meds available, I'll give them. With these ones, I seem to have a pretty good "mental clock" to know when the next dose is available. 2nd night, B bed arrives—another pain management person. I do what I can for her, she eventually goes to sleep. Through the night A bed is fine, actually seemed relaxed that night. In the morning, I hear A bed tell B bed that I'm a good nurse and will take care of her. I work nights, so I know planning is easier for stuff like that, and I can make myself more available than during days when the phones won't stop ringing.

Other patients, like a woman that had gone blind and had MS and was increasingly weaker. She was pretty needy and slow, but I learned how she liked things. I could generally sense her being more at ease when she knew I was her nurse. Some people need more time and TLC. Yes, spending 10+ minutes getting her on and off the commode several times/night (basically every 2 hours), but it can just be about helping her keep her dignity. Yes, she swallowed 1 tablet at a time, slowly. She often spoke so softly, I had to put my ear close to hear her. She was needy, she took time, but in the end, she was also the reason I became a nurse.

On the other hand, I have very little tolerance for non-compliant patients (excluding those with psychiatric disorders).

MEDICATIONS

I jokingly refer to all medications as poisons. This is to remind you that ALL medications have side effects, including over-the-counter medications, herbs, and supplements. Of course the risk outweighs the benefits, but drug-drug interactions and adverse responses do happen. When your patient develops a new condition, look at the meds you are giving them first. Prolonged QT? Probably due to one of the meds they're on. New rash on their back or chest? Maybe the IV antibiotic you just started.

> I once had a renal patient who had a high potassium level in the absence of any potassium replacement or medication. It was puzzling, because usually when a patient has a high potassium, potassium supplements are the culprit.
>
> Finally, a light bulb came on. This patient, among other things, was on an ace-inhibitor for his blood pressure. Was that the culprit? I asked the nephrologist and he discontinued the ace-inhibitor. Within one day, the potassium was normal.

This is an example of practice-based evidence. From then on, I always looked for ace-inhibitors in my renal patients with hyperkalemia.

NASOGASTRIC TUBES (NGTs)

Placing the nasogastric tube for a short time in ice before inserting makes it stiffer. This helps prevent it from circling on itself and coming out of the mouth.

The key is to sit your patient upright. Look at their nares and pick the one that appears to be the most open. Start to insert and then have them swallow *when the tube hits the back of the throat.* When the swallowing and the pushing are coordinated, it goes in like a dream.

There's something satisfying about getting an NGT in the right spot and getting a flood of stomach contents in return.

OPIOID-INDUCED RESPIRATORY DEPRESSION

End tidal CO2 is an earlier indicator of opioid-induced respiratory depression than is SpO2.

You can have a normal SpO2 and an elevated CO2. This is when the patient is still oxygenated but retaining carbon dioxide. What does an elevated CO2 mean? CO2 retention is caused by not exhaling. It means they are not breathing enough. Wake them up, stimulate them, tell them to take big breaths.

The first sign of respiratory depression in a patient receiving opioids is sedation. This is before any other metrics. Treat the patient, not the machine. Your patient may be drowsy but alert when wakened, but they may be so sleepy they fall asleep while talking. In this case, turn off the PCA (if they are on one) and hold narcotics until you've consulted with the provider. Some hospitals use the POSS scale (Pasero Opioid-induced Sedation Scale) to assess patients on opioids for sedation, but if not, simply assess how sedated they are.

Note: Don't confuse the RASS (Richmond-Agitation Sedation Scale) with the POSS. The RASS scale is another sedation scale mostly used in ICU to assess sedation. The difference between the RASS and the POSS is that the RASS is used for intentional sedation, while the POSS is used to measure unintentional sedation induced by opioids.

OXYGEN DELIVERY DEVICES

It's important to know your most commonly used oxygen delivery devices.

- Nasal cannula. Most frequently used oxygen delivery device. Delivers FIO2 of up to 40% at a flow rate of commonly 2–5 L/minute, can be used at up to 8 L/minute. Be sure and point curved nasal prongs downwards, not upwards.
- Hi-flow nasal cannula. Delivers FIO2 of 50% to 75% at a flow rate of up to 60 L/minute.
- Simple mask. Used to deliver oxygen at a higher flow rate than nasal cannulas. Sometimes you can take a mask off for meals and replace it for a short time with a nasal cannula, keeping an eye on their 02 saturation, and closely watching how it's tolerated. Remember, always treat the patient, not the machine! Can deliver a concentration of 35% to 50% at 5–10 L/minute.
- Non-rebreather mask. Non-rebreathers have an attached reservoir bag semi-inflated with oxygen and are designed to prevent inhalation of room air or exhaled air. Delivers 60% to 80% oxygen at 8–10 L/minute into the reservoirs bag.
- Venturi mask. Delivers a specific amount of air and oxygen. Typically, can be set at and deliver 24, 28, 31, 35 and 40% oxygen.
- Humidifiers. Can be attached to any oxygen delivery device. Some patients are very sensitive to air flow and can get bloody noses from "dry" air. Humidifiers are recommended on nasal cannulas at 4 L/minute and higher.

You can see that the above devices are used in progression according to the patient's need for oxygen. Know where your devices are located on your par wall. Since respiratory distress situations can happen rapidly, it's important that you can grab a device from the supply room without wasted search time.

PCTs AND CNAs

Befriend your non-licensed personnel. The PCTs or nursing assistants on your unit can make or break you. They are the heart of patient care and a good nursing assistant makes all the difference in a patient's stay. Most of them have hearts of gold and are some of the hardest working people you will ever meet. One nursing assistant I know quietly worked two jobs and put both her children through prestigious medical schools.

As a new nurse, the PCTs/nursing assistants are watching to see how you treat them. They particularly resent the registered nurse who implies that some tasks are beneath her. An example is the nurse in the patient's room who calls the nursing assistant when the patient asks for a bedpan instead of simply putting them on the bedpan when she has the time to do so. Don't be that nurse.

Most PCTs/nursing assistants will do anything for you once you show you have no problem jumping in to help clean up a patient or make up a bed. It's really about showing them respect. When I was a new nurse and worked Ortho, there was a nursing assistant named Annabelle who taught me most of what I know about orthopedic patients. She taught me how to turn a post-op hip replacement safely and get them up to a chair for meals. My entire career I've been grateful to Annabelle.

The problem is that you can't always jump in and help out. You can be drowning, and a patient asks you for a cup of coffee. The best thing to do is not to stop and fetch coffee when you really are drowning. It's to delegate to your PCT or nursing assistant. You can do everything a PCT or nursing assistant can do, but a PCT or nursing assistant can't admit a patient or start a blood transfusion for you.

The key is to do what you can and call your PCT/nursing assistant when you have to. Once they know you are willing to help them when you can, they will understand when you can't.

Mutual Respect

I have a lot of regard for other non-licensed staff, such as housekeepers. They are often forgotten when appreciation is handed out and overlooked for what they contribute. Acknowledge them and show your appreciation. Everyone's contribution is needed and important.

PHONE NUMBERS, KEY

You may have a badge buddy with a list of key phone numbers. There are some numbers you will call so often that you will soon memorize them. At a minimum, have these numbers memorized:

- Code or RRT
- Pharmacy
- Distribution or Materials Management
- Key providers
- Charge Nurse

Some hospitals have numbers to call for a sepsis alert, STEMI alert, and so on. The operator has a phone tree and will call the affected departments. For example, in a stroke alert, the operator will notify diagnostic imaging so they can clear the CT table for the incoming patient.

POTASSIUM REPLACEMENT

When you are replacing potassium, it is much more efficacious to give oral potassium than IV potassium (practice-based evidence). You may not find a pharmacist or doctor to agree with you, but any experienced nurse will agree, and pharmacists and doctors don't administer potassium, nurses do. So if your patient can tolerate oral potassium and you have a choice, don't hesitate.

It is also more difficult to raise the potassium when the magnesium level is low, so check your patient's magnesium level when they are hypokalemic.

SEPSIS

When caring for a post-op patient, if they have an elevated temp or white count, think lungs, bladder, wound, pneumonia, UTI, or surgical wound infection. Know that a drop in temperature and a drop in white count can be an early sign of sepsis. Early detection is key to preventing complications and death.

SERVICE RECOVERY

An important skill set is service recovery. Patients or customers who experience service recovery are even more loyal than customers who've never had a bad experience or service recovery.

Service recovery is needed when something's gone wrong or the patient perceives that something has gone wrong. When a person feels unfairly wronged, they expect extreme apology and atonement. This is true of everyone.

It's okay to apologize when a patient feels wronged. Apologizing does not mean there was wrongdoing. Saying "I'm sorry that happened" does not convey agreement, just acknowledgment. You can empathize, "I wouldn't want anyone else to have that same experience."

Never argue. Telling a patient that "it's the policy" will not help matters. Likewise, telling a doctor that "it's policy for you to sign the restraint order" is not going to be helpful. It takes two to escalate a situation. Things will not escalate unless you push back, so remain calm.

If your patient is highly emotional, ask "What can I do for you now?" to switch them over to a cognitive state from an emotional state.

Notify your charge nurse or supervisor so they can help. It's important to let nurse managers know of patient complaint situations because they do not want to be blind-sided without having any prior knowledge of the event. A classic example is a nurse manager coming to work on a Monday morning and getting a call from administration about a problem that occurred on her unit over the weekend.

Your nurse manager would rather receive a text from you on the weekend than be taken by surprise Monday morning.

SUPPLY ROOM

Familiarize yourself with key supplies in the supply room. Know that supplies used every day are stocked in the supply room, while supplies that are used infrequently or are too bulky to stock on the floor on a par wall are housed off the unit in materials management, sometimes called distribution or the warehouse. Materials management is used for single use products, whereas central supply is a separate department that sterilizes and re-packages reusable supplies and equipment such as procedural trays with instruments.

Next time you go to work, find out where you would obtain a thoracentesis tray if needed.

Especially teach yourself where to quickly find key supplies commonly called for in an emergency so you won't panic and fumble.

- Connection tubing. Used to connect a device to wall suction, such as NGT tubes, PureWick external catheters, or chest drainage systems.
- Oxygen delivery devices
- IV start kits or supplies

TAP WATER ENEMAS

If you have a patient scheduled for a colonoscopy or sigmoidoscopy, you will have orders to prep until clear. A common mistake is to stop administering the enemas before the results are clear. In this case, the procedure might be delayed, or at the least, you'll have invoked the wrath of the GI nurses and doctors. Clear means clear. Hang the enema fluid high. Reach your arm straight up above your head as far as it will go. That is how high.

- Roll the patient side to side until well mixed.
- Do not fear giving repeat enemas. No, they will *not* get water intoxication. You are not done until it is clear. Okay, maybe tinted but essentially clear.

I speak from experience having worked a short time in the GI Lab. It is frustrating for the doctors and nurses when patients arrive from the floors insufficiently prepped. The reason for ordering enemas till clear is that the doctor cannot visualize the bowel properly if there is still fecal material in the bowels.

I found that many times, the PCTs or nursing assistants administer the enemas. If so, you must ask to see the results before they are flushed to determine if they are clear. Again, water intoxication from pre-procedure enemas is not a concern.

VISITORS

You will be the first to notice that some visitors wear your patient out. Your patient may be bright and perky while their visitors are there, but then be utterly exhausted when they leave. This is especially true for those patients who try to entertain their visitors and for visitors who are not particularly sensitive.

Patients are usually the last to complain that their visitors are exhausting, and instead just collapse when they leave. In the past I have made a pact with patients to come in after the visitors have been there a certain amount of time, say, thirty minutes, and apologetically shoo them out. In this way I was the bad guy.

There's nothing wrong with family at the bedside, but there's a difference between a quiet, attentive family member and a loud group.

Sometimes a family member will want you to give them permission to leave. They may feel guilty and feel they have to stay at the bedside 24/7. It can be helpful to let them know the best thing they can do for their loved one is to take care of themselves; go home, shower, change clothes, take a nap. They will need their energy for when their loved one is discharged home. You can take their number, make sure they know your name, and promise to call them if anything changes. Let them know you are accessible, and that they can call you as well.

CHAPTER 7

SAFE PRACTITIONER

Making a medication error is devastating. It can cause you to question your competency and even your decision to be a nurse. When a medication error causes harm, it causes moral distress for the nurse and is linked to second victim syndrome.

After a nurse makes a medication error, they can feel guilty, embarrassed, depressed, and fearful of making another error. Some nurses even choose to leave the profession. You, too, will make mistakes because we are only human, but the important thing is to realize you are not alone and to work through it. Working through it means to experience the feelings, which can be overwhelming. Talk to someone. Identify exactly how the mistake occurred and correct your practice to safeguard against future mistakes.

JoAnne was administering a Pronestyl drip to her cardiac patient. The doctor came in and placed the patient on an oral antiarrhythmic with orders to discontinue the IV Pronestyl drip. Much later that day, the patient coded, and during the code, JoAnne looked up to see that the Pronestyl was still running. She immediately realized her mistake. She had intended to discontinue the drip but got distracted and forgot. The patient died, and JoAnne chose to never work another day as a nurse.

My own first medication error resulted in severe disciplinary action but also ultimately in deep reflection which made me a better nurse. You can read my experience under "I Was Suspended" on my blog, nursecode.com.

Adults learn from making mistakes. When training preceptors, I encourage them to let residents discover their own mistakes when possible for that very reason. This should only be done when there is no serious danger to a patient.

A common mistake every nurse makes, and you will, too, takes place when hanging an antibiotic on a patient who has a primary IV going, such as D51/2. The nurse spikes the antibiotic, primes the secondary tubing, and hangs the antibiotic properly above the level of the primary IV. They program the pump for the correct infusion rate and time of infusion. They walks away, satisfied their task is complete.

Later they return, glance up at the antibiotic bag and see it is still full. What? On second glance, they see that the roller clamp is still clamped. They are shocked but never make that mistake again.

CAUSES OF MISTAKES

There are all kinds of valid reasons we make mistakes, and it's good to know what they are so you can be aware of times when you are more susceptible to making an error.

Distractions and Interruptions

All too often nurses are interrupted during medication administration.

Many years ago, the well-known error of a nurse who inadvertently drank chloral hydrate was reported to the Institute for Safe Medication Practices (ISMP). She poured chloral hydrate, a sleeping medication, into a medicine cup and walked down the hall to administer it. On the way she was interrupted by a provider, and while deep in conversation, lifted it to her mouth and drank it as if it were coffee. It was in her coffee hand, she was chatting, and her brain was on autopilot. She had to be driven home to sleep it off.

Multitasking

Multitasking is not a value, and the word is a misnomer. Cognitive stacking is a better, more descriptive term. There is no such thing as safe multitasking when it comes to medication administration.

Imagine that you are driving a car with patients as your passengers. You would not drive and text or try to follow complex GPS instructions while simultaneously listening to a podcast.

Following the Institute of Medicine's (IOM) recommendation, some hospitals have established a no interruption or distraction-free zone around the automated drug dispensing cabinet. Some hospitals have nurses wear a colored vest while passing medications.

Follow your hospital's procedure but even if there is no official distraction-free policy, make one around yourself. Doctors are not interrupted during surgery. Pilots are not interrupted during takeoff, but nurses are commonly interrupted when administering highly dangerous medications. Refuse to be distracted. Visitors and staff can be educated to hold their questions, allowing you to concentrate on safe medication administration.

It is okay to say, "I'm passing meds right now and I can find that out for you as soon as I'm finished."

Alarm Fatigue

We are all subject to lapses in concentration, fatigue, or distraction. Alarm fatigue occurs when you are exposed to multiple alarms and frequent alarms. It's really sensory overload, and it leads to desensitization because most alarms are false or otherwise non-actionable alarms.

One thing you can do to reduce a common alarm is to change your monitored patients' electrodes daily. This reduces the nuisance alarms generated by electrodes not adhering properly. Also customize the parameters on alarms such as heart rate alarms, so the alarm will be meaningful.

Inattentional Blindness

Inattentional blindness is when we complete tasks reflexively or on autopilot. When on autopilot, our brains do not process what our eyes see.

> I once drove through a red light when driving home at midnight after working sixteen hours straight. The only reason I knew was because of the flashing red lights in my rear view mirror. The minute I saw the flashing lights I realized what I'd done, but it wasn't intentional. I pulled over and the police officer leaned in and said, "Did you know you just ran a red light?" The happy ending to my story is that he saw my stethoscope laying on the seat and said "I hate giving nurses tickets. I might see you in the ED someday! But take this as a warning, okay?"

Inattentional blindness happens when you drive home and don't remember how you got there. It happens when a person takes their daily dose of medication or birth control pills or vitamins and minutes later can't recall if they took them. Did they take the birth control pill today or was that yesterday?

A well-known example of inattentional blindness is when a group of radiologists were given an X-ray and asked to look for signs of cancer. Several of them did not recognize that the patient was missing a collarbone. Another example of inattentional blindness is the well-known YouTube video *selective attention test*, in which a gorilla that appears on the screen is not noticed by the viewer because they are too focused on the task given to them at the start of the video: counting the number of times a basketball is passed among a group of people.

A patient with a nasal cannula returned from X-ray and was transferred back to bed by the transport team. Shortly afterwards, she began to show signs of respiratory distress. Several clinicians gathered in the room as she became progressively worse. The nurse went to turn the oxygen flowrate up and noticed the oxygen tubing was connected to the medical air outlet and not the oxygen outlet. This whole time, the patient had not received oxygen.

The patient in the above example was my patient. Was it me? Did I connect the oxygen tubing to the air outlet while I was on auto-pilot? Did the transport person do it, or my CNA? I don't know, but I could have. We are all capable of mistakes when we're not mindful. The opposite of inattentional blindness is mindfulness and keeping your brain alert at all times during your shift.

Bias of Authority

Speak up if you have questions about an order. In 2018, fatally high doses of Fentanyl were given to over 25 ICU patients at Mount Carmel hospital in Columbus, Ohio.

The prescribing doctor was charged with manslaughter, but there are nurses and pharmacists who were also complicit and investigated. Many of the nurses were new, and when they asked the doctor about the dose (as high as 500–2000 micrograms), he authoritatively gave an answer that satisfied them enough to administer up to a hundred times the usual dose of Fentanyl.

Bias of authority also occurs between nurses. Unfortunately, some nurses will give an incorrect answer rather than say "I don't know." You can be given wrong information this way. As a newly licensed nurse, it's important to learn who is credible. It is your nursing practice and you are responsible, whether a doctor, nurse, or a pharmacist gives you wrong information.

For example, just because a nurse is a charge nurse does not mean she is credible. But because of their title, charge nurses carry a bias of authority.

Jenifer asked her charge nurse to independently check her heparin drip rate calculation. Jenifer got one answer, but the charge nurse got a different answer. Rather than reconcile the answers, Jenifer assumed the charge nurse must be right and she must be wrong. As a result, Jenifer overdosed the patient, which contributed to a femoral bleed.

In reality, the charge nurse had not managed a heparin drip for years and was distracted when asked. The right thing to do would have been for both to independently recalculate the rate until their answers reconciled.

Use your hospital-approved resources, such as Lippincott, to check how to do procedures, and always refer to policy. Your educator is a good resource and will help guide you in the right direction.

Variance

Varying from routine can lead to error.

A tragic example of how variance causes error is in the case of the nurse practitioner who usually did not take her daughter to childcare, as her husband did. That fateful day, her husband was sick and she drove their child to childcare. Or she intended to. The baby was in the car seat in the back and the mother drove to work, parked, and left her child in the car. She returned eight hours later to find her dead daughter.

The way to prevent medication errors and safeguard against error is to do things the same way every time. For example, scan the patient's armband, scan the medication, administer the medication to the patient, then document as given. Never vary and always perform these steps in the same order. Performing these steps out of order will eventually result in errors of omission or overdose.

Checklists and Timeouts

Reduction of variance is the reason for the growth in the use of checklists and timeouts in healthcare. There is a science to the safety of checklists. Pilots, co-pilots, and air traffic controllers follow a precision pre-takeoff checklist regardless of how many times they've performed the procedure. Flight aviation checklists are intended to ensure that everything is done and no steps are missed. Likewise, standardized pre-op checklists have been found to be helpful during patient handoff, before surgery, and at discharge, when there are multiple steps.

According to the Joint Commission, a timeout is when the entire surgical team pauses immediately before the procedure to confirm the correct patient, procedure, and site. Timeouts before surgery and procedures are required as part of the Universal Protocol to reduce errors.

When you are out of routine for any reason, you are at risk for making an error. Variance causes errors and operating from a routine helps to prevent errors.

Normalization of Deviance

Shortcuts and drifts in practice can lead to normalization of deviance. Normalization of deviance is when deviating from policy or procedure happens so frequently that it becomes the norm.

> Normalization of deviance caused newly licensed nurse Sara to make a serious error. The patient was ordered to receive Nimotop and Sara had observed her preceptor giving it. Nimotop comes in a gel capsule with liquid inside. Sara had watched her preceptor pierce the capsule and draw up the content in a syringe, remove the needle tip, and squirt the contents in the patient's mouth.
>
> Sara carefully pierced the capsule, drew up the medication with a syringe and then injected it into the IV port. Her brain automatically associated a syringe in her hand with IV administration. As soon as Sara started to push the medication, she knew she had done something wrong. She withdrew the syringe and tearfully got her preceptor. Fortunately, the patient did not suffer any lasting effects.

Holding a syringe in her hand triggered Sara to administer an IV injection. The root cause of the problem was using a syringe intended for IV use for oral administration.

Confirmation Bias

Confirmation bias is when you see what you expect to see. It's what happened in 2007 to the nurse who gave the newborn twins of actor Dennis Quaid one thousand times the common dosage of a blood thinner. The heparin vials contained 10,000 units of heparin per mL instead of 10 units per mL.

A similar mistake happened to nurse Kimberly Hiatt, a fifty-year-old longtime critical care nurse at Seattle Children's Hospital, who died by suicide from second victim syndrome seven months after accidentally overdosing a fragile baby.

In the fall of 2010, Kimberly Hiatt, a highly regarded and experienced nurse, received an order to administer 140 milligrams of calcium chloride IV to her patient, a nine-month-old.

Kimberly expected to see a vial with 10 milligrams per mL. Instead the label read 100 milligrams of calcium chloride per mL. She administered 1.4 grams of calcium chloride instead of 140 milligrams. Hours later the baby went into tachycardia and a serum level of calcium chloride was ordered. Abnormally high levels were revealed, and the baby died five days later.

It was not determined that the overdose was a clear cause of death as the baby was frail and had severe heart problems, but Kimberly Hiatt was a second victim of this tragic mistake.

At Vanderbilt hospital, a nurse gave Vecuronium (a paralytic) instead of Versed (a sedative) to a seventy-five-year-old female patient going for a PET scan. RaDonda Vaught typed "ve" into the search field of the automatic med dispensing cabinet (ADC) and it quickly populated with drug names, "vecuronium" being at the top of the list. Versed was not listed because it was listed in the drug library as midazolam. RaDonda took out the wrong drug and administered it to her patient, then left, thinking she had given Versed. The woman died from suffocation.

There are several takeaways from the RaDonda Vaught story, but one to keep in mind is to be mindful when using the "override" function in your automatic drug dispensing cabinet. There are legitimate reasons for choosing "override" but once you do that, any built-in safeguards are no longer enabled.

Connections and Workarounds

Medical device connections are a prime cause of error. Cases reported to the FDA include the case of an obstetric nurse who connected a bag of pain medication intended for an epidural catheter to the mother's intravenous (IV) line, resulting in a fatal cardiac arrest. Other cases involved IV tubing mistakenly connected to a trach cuff port in a pediatric patient and IV tubing erroneously connected to a nasal cannula.

To ensure safety, manufacturers of enteral devices have standardized connections to avoid accidental connections between enteral and non-enteral tubing.

Be on alert anytime you connect one tube to another. There are devices called Christmas trees and other graduated connectors that allow you to connect two tubes that do not otherwise fit. There are legitimate uses for connectors, but it should be a red flag when you are attempting to connect tubes that do not fit and perhaps were not intended to be connected.

Increased workloads and poor design can lead to taking shortcuts. Nurses are famous for workarounds or "MacGyvering" skills. Workarounds are when frontline clinicians bypass policy and safety procedures, often because nurses are figuring out how to get the work done in time with a lack of resources.

These are all examples of how nurses working in chaotic environments under pressure with multiple competing distractions are subject to making mistakes of inattentional blindness, confirmation bias, bias of authority, errors of variance, and normalization of deviance.

The point is, don't underestimate how easy it is for even experienced clinicians to make an error. The healthcare industry is often encouraged to be as safe as the airline industry, citing strict takeoff and landing protocols. The difference is that pilots and co-pilots don't have call lights going off and visitors and doctors interrupting them during takeoff. Our environment is much more chaotic, and we have to be vigilant at all times.

Key Tips for Safe Medication Administration

- Check for patient allergies every time you administer a medication.
- Follow the six rights: right patient, right medication, right dose, right time, right route, right documentation.
- Know the reversal agents of the medications you are administering. What is the reversal agent for heparin? What is the reversal agent for opioids, and what is the reversal agent for benzodiazepines? Look these up and commit them to memory.
- Perform independent double checks mindfully. Double checks requiring a math calculation should be conducted independently, not with one nurse doing the math and the other nurse looking on.
- Listen to patients who question their medications. If a patient asks, "What is this brown pill? I don't usually take it," double check the order and the indication.

- Be very careful when using the override function in automated drug dispensing cabinets, such as Pyxis or Omnicell.
- Never get so comfortable and confident that you think you can't make a mistake.

PATIENT FALLS

Patient falls, along with pressure injuries, nosocomial infections such as ventilator associated pneumonia (VAP), catheter associated urinary tract infections (CAUTIs), and central line associated blood stream infections (CLABSIs), are nursing-sensitive indicators. Nursing-sensitive indicators reflect the outcomes of nursing care. They are outcomes under our control, as nurses, that affect patients.

Patient falls are a huge concern in hospitals. Patient falls can be prevented by purposeful hourly rounding and by being in tune with your patient's needs.

In ten years as a nurse manager investigating falls, I can say that most falls are caused by patients having to go the bathroom. The urgency to urinate or defecate is powerful and drives patients out of bed. They may be on sedating medication, have tubes attached, and may not be familiar with the room layout. By the time the bed alarm sounds, the patient can be on the floor.

Meaningful hourly rounding is the best way to prevent patient falls. It is not enough to ask a patient "Do you want to go to the bathroom?" but instead say "I have the time, let's go to the bathroom now."

In the same spirit, ask open-ended questions rather than close-ended questions. Asking "What questions do you have?" (open-ended) when providing patient education is different than asking "Do you have any questions?" (close-ended).

Close-ended questions prompt for a yes or no answer, and most people will usually give a socially polite answer such as "No, I'm good."

KNOW YOUR POLICIES

Become a policy-driven nurse. It's amazing to me when I ask a nurse to pull up a policy and it's apparent that they've never done it before.

Following policies protects you, your job, your license, and your patients.

> Jon admitted a patient to the ED from a skilled nursing facility who was subsequently admitted to the med-surg unit with pneumonia. He wasn't aware of the policy that said two nurses must perform a skin assessment together. It turned out the patient had a Stage 3 pressure injury. The pressure injury was discovered on hospital day two, which means it most likely was present on admission. Two days is typically not long enough to develop a Stage 3 injury. Because it was not identified on admission, the hospital was responsible for the injury and penalized for the event.

Policies protect patients.

> Lynda catheterized a patient on admission and sent a urine sample for testing because where she previously worked, it was standard procedure. When she entered the order, she selected "standing order" and the order routed to the attending physician for electronic signature. The physician refused to sign the order because he did not order the test. At Lynda's present facility, there

is no standing order to obtain a urine sample for UA and culture when initially inserting a catheter. So now Lynda is in the position of having ordered a test insurance does not have to pay for.

Policies protect nurses, but you have to know what they say.

JUST CULTURE

Fortunately, many facilities have adopted a just culture that encourages nurses to report errors and near misses. A just culture is one of shared accountability where it's understood that mistakes usually occur as a result of system failures. It encourages transparency over secrecy and values learning from mistakes.

FLOATING TO OTHER UNITS

Once you're off of orientation, you should be oriented to any and all units you'll be required to float to. Your competencies need to match the needs of the patients you are assigned to. So for example, if you are floated to ICU and you normally work med-surg, an appropriate assignment might be caring for a patient who is due to be transferred out to med-surg, but not the patient who is on titratable vasopressors.

Ask if there is a policy on floating. Some hospitals do not float newly graduated nurses for a year after they start.

The hospital has an obligation to orient you, and you have an obligation to speak up and ask for help when you are performing a procedure or doing anything for the first time. It's your nursing practice.

GETTING YOUR OWN INSURANCE

Insurance is important because you can be sued even if you did not make a mistake. The hospital will provide their own attorneys if there is a lawsuit against the hospital and you are named, but many cases are not litigated until long after the event. What if you are employed by another facility by that time and your interests are at odds with your employer's? The employer will put their interest before those of an employee, even more so an ex-employee.

While your employer will cover you as long as you were acting within the scope of your license and employment, your employer's insurance may have gaps. If you have your own malpractice insurance, you can hire a lawyer of your choosing.

Some nurses say that they don't want to get insurance because once it's discovered that you have your own insurance, you can be targeted by people who believe you have deep pockets. But discovery cannot take place until you are named as a defendant.

DEFENSIVE CHARTING AND RED FLAGS

You have a tremendous amount of charting to do every day. With time, you will begin to identify situations and people that raise red flags for you. Visitors who carry notepads and write down everything you say may be doing it for their own memory. They may also be prepping for a lawsuit. Red flag.

If a patient fell or had a near fall or assisted fall, that patient is already a risk. Patients who fall once have already proven they fall, and that means they might fall again. Red flag.

With patients where there are red flags for any reason, I take the time to chart more thoroughly. While many hospitals discourage free text, there is always a place to make a note for information not included in the check charting if necessary.

When calling a doctor who says "okay, just keep an eye on it" instead of ordering the scan you anticipated, be sure and note "Doctor notified of patient's change of condition. No orders given."

If you are ever called to testify or give a deposition, your charting will be available to you, and your words will jog your memory.

CHAPTER 8

CRITICAL THINKING

CRITICAL THINKING

Critical thinking, clinical judgment, and problem-solving are among the higher-level skills you will be developing this year. Clinical judgement is a function of critical thinking and problem-solving.

Nurses who are critical thinkers are analytical and curious. The best critical thinkers are full of questions because they are always seeking to understand, recognize patterns, and form rationalizations.

For example, if a patient has low magnesium, you replace the magnesium. That reflects your knowledge that hypomagnesemia should be corrected, and your skill of doing it. But this would also trigger the intellectual curiosity of a nurse with critical thinking. That nurse will search for the underlying cause of the hypomagnesemia.

Critical thinking is stepping back to look at the whole picture. Nurses who are successful critical thinkers are:

- Inquisitive about their work and surroundings
- Sure to gather and collect evidence and pertinent information
- Analytical and self-confident in their own reasoning
- Able to self-reflect

CONTROLLING ANXIETY

What does controlling anxiety have to do with critical thinking? Controlling anxiety is key to becoming a critical thinker. Your anxiety prevents you from hearing and processing what is taking place. Essentially, nurses with high anxiety do not learn well. When intense enough, anxiety is disabling. If you have disabling anxiety, make an appointment with your provider to see if treatment is right for you.

There are different levels and intensities of anxiety. There will be times and situations where you have overwhelming anxiety and feel unprepared and inadequate to meet all the competing demands on your time and energy. Usually it's when you have a change in patient condition or an emergency, but it can just be an overwhelming shift.

You may also experience anxiety after your shift wondering if you attended to all your tasks and documented everything. To some degree, all nurses experience anxiety and even have dreams about forgetting something. This is common and normal, even in experienced nurses.

When you begin to feel anxious on the job, take a deep breath in and a deep breath out. Remind yourself that you can only do one thing at a time. Now you have to pick which one, based on patient safety. Prioritizing and having a plan helps you manage your anxiety because then you are channeling some of your energy productively. Having a plan helps you to feel in control, whereas feeling powerless exacerbates anxiety.

It's always helpful to bounce your plan off your preceptor or a trusted colleague.

"My patient is GI bleeding and I've put a call in to the doctor. My plan is to start another IV. He has one but he's on an amiodarone drip, so if the doctor orders blood, I'll be ready with IV access. I've already checked with the blood bank and he has two units screened, but not cross-matched. I'll check to see if he has a consent for blood transfusion signed—if not, the doctor will have to explain the risks and benefits. Is this a good plan?"

Your preceptor may add some helpful feedback, such as, *"Have a current set of vital signs ready and make sure to check to see if he's on any anticoagulants."*

PRIORITIZING

Your workflow will improve once you become faster at your tasks. Structure, as in setting priorities, reduces anxiety. You have to be able to set priorities in order to survive. Initially you will prioritize according to your scheduled tasks. As you gain experience, you will prioritize according to the changing conditions of your patients. It's a shift from nurse-centered practice to patient-centered practice. See more on prioritizing in Chapter 2, What to Expect from Your Orientation, under Time Management.

RECOGNIZING ABNORMAL

Critical thinking means recognizing abnormalities and then assigning meaning to what you recognized. It's easier to identify abnormal signs and symptoms in case studies or in simulation lab than in real life. In textbooks you're given normal ranges and abnormal ranges. The problem is that patients haven't read the book and don't follow the algorithms. Just yesterday, a colleague showed me a strip of a patient in a third degree heart block with a rate of 60 bpm. This is fast for a third degree block. You have to keep an open mind and consider all possibilities.

What textbooks don't teach you is that it's not just a matter of normal or abnormal, it's what's normal or abnormal for your particular patient. A change from baseline is clinically significant. If a patient is normally very animated and talkative and now is withdrawn and quiet, that is noteworthy, even in the presence of normal vital signs. Look for the cause. Did their doctor just deliver bad news? Are they in pain? Some people become very quiet when in pain. Is this a change in level of consciousness? Context is key. You as the nurse have intimate clinical knowledge of the patient.

Recognizing significant abnormalities in patients takes seeing both many normalities and abnormalities in patients with many conditions and in many situations.

For example, how is a new nurse to know what normal looks like in a patient just transferred out from recovery room after surgery? You may recognize vital signs that are outside of the normal parameters but fail to grasp the meaning. This is normal. Your clinical judgment will develop once you have had sufficient experience to compare multiple patient responses. Interpreting the significance of abnormal findings is a skill that comes with clinical experience.

Michael was admonished by his preceptor because he failed to recognize a change in condition in his post-op patient. Michael had received back only one post-op patient to date, the one under question. The patient appeared to be sedated, but since the post-op nurse helped transfer the patient to bed without concern, Michael thought it must be normal. As it turns out, the patient was overly-sedated from narcotics given in the recovery room and became even more sedated within a few minutes of being put to bed. When the preceptor came in the room, she recognized the signs of sedation and the context. The preceptor immediately gave naloxone (Narcan), a reversal agent for opioids, and proceeded to chastise Michael.

In talking with the manager and the resident later, it was clear to me that Michael had no baseline for comparison. As he explained, "I thought that was how someone coming out of surgery is supposed to look." He took his cue from the recovery room nurse, who was unconcerned. It is natural to rely on the judgment of more experienced clinicians.

Likewise, recognizing a patient with sepsis takes experience.

Once I came to work and was walking past room 4124. It was 0700 and the patient, Carol, a 37-year-old, was lying in bed. Still walking, I glanced at her bedside monitor and it showed a heart rate of 108. I stopped.

Going in the room, I dropped my purse down on top of the linen hamper knowing it was a violation of infection control standards, but I needed my hands free and there was no other surface area. I had a sense of overriding urgency. I looked at her closely. Something was very wrong. She was awake but a little drowsy with her left hand bandaged in a bulky dressing and elevated to an IV pole. I called for a set of vitals while her night nurse filled me in on her history. She had been camping with her family over the weekend at the beach. At some point she stuck her hand in a pile of wood and was bitten by a spider. Within 24 hours, it was red and swollen with red streaks darting up her arm. Her temp was 97.6 and her blood pressure 106 over 52.

I called ICU to see if they had a bed because I knew she was not stable. They did have a bed, so I called her doctor and said, "Your patient really doesn't look good, she needs to go to ICU" and we had her transferred to ICU within ten minutes. Before change of shift report.

What was it that alarmed me just walking by the room and why was her nurse not alarmed? A heart rate of 108 in a 37-year-old woman who is resting in bed is enough to investigate. Combined with a source of infection, she was probably septic.

I've since thought about the nurse's responsibility. I was a manager at the time and felt responsible for all the care given on the unit. But the nurse did not have enough experience to know that a heart rate of 108 was a red flag given the context. What I did expect from the nurse was to at least question "Why would a patient have a heart rate of 108 just lying in bed?" and "Why is the patient's temp 97.6 (also a sign of sepsis)?"

There is an addition to my spider story.

Fast forward twenty years. I was teaching a basic life support class to nursing students and was telling my story. The point of the story was, "Treat the patient, not the machine." After all, a heart rate of 108 in and of itself and without context is not particularly alarming. I told the class that I didn't really know the outcome, because as with most cases, I didn't follow every patient who transferred to ICU. There were always other brightly burning fires to attend to. After I told my story, a nursing student in class raised her hand and quietly said, "That was my mother you took care of. Carol. She died in the ICU."

That was really sad to hear, and reminded me what a small world it is, and what a small community nursing is. Truth is stranger than fiction.

A NOTE ON INTUITION

You may hear experienced nurses urge you to "listen to your gut." You may not understand what they are talking about or you may think, "Oh, no, I've got nothing! What does that even mean?" The problem is that you have not yet developed sufficient assessment skills or experienced enough problem situations to the point where you have meaningful gut feelings. What you likely feel, if anything, is a generalized anxiety more than a focused meaningful sense that something specifically is wrong with your patient.

Tiffany, an experienced nurse, was at the nurses' station and glanced up. She looked across the hall directly into the room and saw the face of the patient lying in bed. Something in what she saw made her drop the chart in her hand and dash to the room. At that exact same moment, a newly licensed nurse, Michael, walked by the room, glanced in, and kept walking without breaking his stride. What did Tiffany see that Michael did not see? I call it "The Look," but that is not helpful to you. It was a certain slackness in facial tone, perhaps, a paleness of color, a pallor. All Tiffany knew was that he was about to arrest. Tiffany had seen enough patients at time of arrest to know and recognize the signs.

Intuition is not some mystical skill that good nurses have. It's a function of analyzing and synthesizing while drawing on past experience all done at superfast speed and without conscious reasoning. Your intuition will develop later with experiential learning. Intuition comes with pattern recognition over time as with the patient who has "The Look" and is about to code. It takes years of observation and experience. You will hear experienced nurses say, "she looks really sick."

Nurses who say patients "don't look good" or "they're really sick" and can't really explain it further except as intuition are really synthesizing cues. Doctors understand this as well, and come to trust experienced nurses who say, "I can't put my finger on it, the vital signs are okay, but your patient really looks sick."

This is not intended to discourage you; it's to confirm that you need time and clinical exposure. You most likely look at skilled competent nurses and think "I'll never be like them," but you will. They were once like you, and you will someday be like them. Remember, chances are that student nurses on your floor are already looking at you and wishing they could be like you!

So, when a nurse says to you, "trust your gut," just nod and realize it is well-intentioned but a premature expectation. It's not something you can aspire to or study for. Do follow this—when something doesn't seem right to you, pay attention and ask for help.

Trusting your gut is a result of growth. Reading previous nurse's assessments and notes will help you, as will reading doctor's progress notes.

ANTICIPATE

Critical thinkers anticipate the next step.

Some of the best advice I can share with you is to be prepared. Be in a state of anticipation, meaning always anticipate the worst that could happen.

Jason went to pull a sheath with his preceptor.

His preceptor pulled him aside and said, "Jason, before we go in the room, you need to think through the worst that can happen and how you'll respond, so you'll be prepared to respond if it happens."

Jason: "Okay, well, I'm going to remove the femoral arterial sheath and hold pressure until it stops bleeding. So the worst that can happen is uncontrolled bleeding."

Preceptor: "Wrong. Bleeding is not the worst that can happen. It's messy, yes, but if they keep bleeding, you keep holding pressure. Eventually it will clot."

Jason: "Oh. Is it a vagal reaction? Where the heart rate slows down?"

Preceptor: "Okay, better. What will you do?"

Jason: "Give Atropine 0.5 mg every three to five minutes up to a max of 3 mg."

Preceptor: "Right. Know how to get it in a hurry or take some in with you to have instantly available. You are on the right track. But that's still not the worst that can happen. The worst that can happen is that the vessel will occlude and that is basically a heart attack. If that happens, we'll call a code and start CPR. But we are going to prevent that from happening by doing our best to prevent a vagal response. And if the patient does vagal, we'll immediately give Atropine."

Likewise, if you are a labor and delivery nurse, be prepared for the worst when you go into every delivery. Think through what steps should be taken if the mother hemorrhages or the fetus has fetal dystocia. Then you will go into an automatic response of doing the right thing because you're prepared.

PREVENTING CODES

There are really very few causes of sudden death—or death without warning—in a hospital. Whenever I hear a code being called overhead, I wonder what may have been missed and if it could have been prevented. According to Wenqi, M., et al (2015, p. 208), "The majority of adverse events are preceded by a period of abnormal vital signs (minutes to hours), which could be identified through consistent and accurate monitoring." But early crucial warnings of change in condition are often missed.

A pulmonary embolism (PE) is one such cause of sudden death. PEs can be fatal, and that's why there is such an emphasis on venous thromboembolism prevention, which is applying your SCDs and administering prophylactic blood thinners.

In the case of a PE, you may not have any warning signs at all. Your post-op patient may be seated, stand up, and suddenly experience the classic signs of PE—chest pain, shortness of breath, diaphoresis.

Aside from PE, other causes of sudden death can include a myocardial infarction (MI), a stroke, or a dissecting abdominal aneurysm.

The point is that before most patients code, they give you ample warning. There are clinical antecedents. That is why early warning scores are important in recognizing sepsis. Prior to an arrest, the patient may have respiratory depression or deterioration in mental function. Do not ignore a patient who was previously verbal suddenly struggling to find words. It could be a stroke, a TIA, or hypoglycemia.

I recall a code called on a patient and asking the monitor tech what rhythm the patient was in. "A third-degree (complete) heart block," she said. I looked at the strip, and sure enough, it was a third-degree block. "But what rhythm was the patient in before the third-degree block? Before she coded?" I asked.

She looked at me strangely. "A sinus rhythm." To this day, I doubt that. I believe the patient was in a Mobitz Type I or a Mobitz Type II, or both, because in my experience patients do not go directly into a third-degree block from a sinus rhythm. There are antecedents and warning that there is pathology at the AV junction. So it's probable the change in rhythm was missed, and definitely critical thinking was lacking in her response.

You will notice that when patients go into V-tach or some other arrhythmia and you tell the provider, they frequently ask, "What rhythm were they in right before?" They will want to see a strip of the beats immediately preceding the arrhythmia. This provides context and clues as to what the abnormal rhythm is. It's always good to be prepared with this information and to start thinking this way yourself.

RESPIRATORY ASSESSMENT

Unfortunately, respiratory rates are often not correctly documented. Nursing assistants and PCTS may not take the time to count the respirations and instead document a guesstimate, falling somewhere within the normal range of 12–16. It's not just nursing assistants and PCTs, though. It's all nurses, and that includes RNs. This is unfortunate because substantial evidence exists that abnormal respiratory rates are a known predictor of serious clinical events.

Vital signs must not only be measured accurately, they must be documented and mindfully assessed by the registered nurse.

Pulse oximetry readings should not be substituted for documenting respiratory rates. SpO2 is not an early indicator of respiratory depression. In fact, the earliest sign of respiratory depression secondary to opiates is level of sedation, followed by elevated CO_2, and finally, decreased SpO2.

CONTEXT: TREAT THE PATIENT,
NOT THE MACHINE

One day I got to work at 0700 and stood behind the monitor tech at the monitor bank, watching forty-eight rhythms of our forty-eight patients march across the screen. The patient in room 4206 had a perfectly paced rhythm—100% AV paced at a rate of 78.

You can imagine the shock when minutes later, the day nursing assistant, who had just come on duty and was rounding to take vital signs, rushed out of room 4206. *"My patient is dead!"* We all ran into the room, and sure enough, the patient was cold, stiff, and clearly dead. How could this be? His rhythm still looked perfect.

A pacemaker will continue to pace when a patient dies. So while the monitor showed a perfect rhythm, the monitor can only show that electrical activity is taking place. It cannot show mechanical activity or that the heart is in fact pumping. That is demonstrated by blood pressure.

Measurements are always interpreted in the context of how the patient presents.

Another time I called the family because their elderly mother had died. She was on telemetry, but was a No Code status, so when she arrested, we did not intervene, and she passed. Her monitor showed asystole. Right after I hung up with the family, she began having a rhythm—wide, bizarre slow beats irregularly marching across the screen at the nurses' station. My patient was alive? And I had just called the family to tell them she was dead? I rushed to the room.

As it turned out, she was having automatic electrical activity that created transient electrical beats on the EKG. She was indeed dead, there was no mechanical activity, and there was no blood pressure. I'm not a country girl, but I understand this is similar to a chicken that runs around after their head is cut off.

Yet another time, working ICU, I was caring for a young man who was dying, and the entire large family was gathered in the room around the bed. As he was actively dying, the eyes of every family member were fixed upwards on the bedside monitor. Every wide bizarre configuration confused them and gave them false hope. I learned that day to turn off the bedside monitor at these times.

PROBLEM SOLVING

Nurses who are critical thinkers are problem-solvers. When you make a clinical decision, always be prepared to speak to your choices, using *safe patient care* as your rationale.

You round on Mrs. Smith and she complains about her IV. On closer inspection, the site is puffy.

Mrs. Smith with the infiltrated IV is most likely going home today. She is eating well and taking fluids. She has no IV meds. Discontinue the IV and go on to do your morning meds on time. Don't waste time restarting the IV. The doctor usually rounds at 0800, wait for him to come rather than call. Time saved.

You are passing morning meds and your patient is scheduled for dialysis.

Following the rules, you would give the antihypertensive medications as ordered because they are on the MAR. As a critical thinker, you realize that dialysis can cause hypotension because a large volume of fluid is being drawn off. Instead call and double-check with the doctor, who may have forgotten to write "hold on day of dialysis."

Your patient is NPO but on a dose of Lantus insulin for the morning.

You may want to automatically hold the insulin, but then you recall that Lantus is a long-acting basal metabolic insulin.

It is not intended to cover food intake but to replace insulin secreted by the pancreas for metabolic function. You call the doctor to confirm if the Lantus should be given or held. The doctor may adjust the dose or give an order to administer the whole dose.

PATTERN RECOGNITION

Pattern recognition comes with a knowledge of the rules and repeated exposure.

It's like a quilt. At first you see somehow pleasing yet random shapes and colors. Then someone with knowledge of quilts points out the pattern, let's say, a log cabin pattern. You learn the pieces and patterns that make up a log cabin pattern. Early log cabin blocks were hand-pieced using strips of fabrics around a central square. In traditional log cabin blocks, one half is made of dark fabrics and the other half light. A red center symbolized the hearth of home and a yellow center represented a welcoming light in the window. You begin to recognize the log cabin pattern in quilts even when the shapes, sizes, and colors are different, but you have to see a lot of log cabin quilts to develop log cabin pattern recognition. Eventually you develop sight recognition, when without looking for the parts (fabric strips around a central square) you recognize the pattern as a log cabin pattern.

Likewise, pattern recognition is in play when you learn basic arrhythmia interpretation. First you learn the rules, then you can begin to recognize patterns when the amplitude or configuration varies. I have nurses all the time who, when shown a strip of A-fib, may be able to identify it as A-fib. But if I ask them to explain their answer they say "Well, it looks like A-fib." So, then I ask, "What are the rules of A-fib?" and they draw a blank. Sight recognition cannot come before learning the rules, because your interpretation will not be accurate when the appearance (rate or amplitude) changes. I tell them A-fib is grossly irregular and has no discernable P wave. Until you've learned and hard-wired the rules, you are not allowed to claim "sight recognition."

JOURNALING

(Journaling is also discussed in Chapter 2: What to Expect from Your Orientation.)

Nurses who are critical thinkers reflect on their own practice.

Journaling is an excellent way to gain critical thinking skills and appreciate your progression. Some days you will become overwhelmed with all the competing demands and feel like you're drowning. This happens to experienced nurses as well.

After an overwhelming shift, write down what happened and what you could have done differently. Try to identify exactly when it was that you lost control.

I had a good morning it started out okay. I was in the middle of passing meds and my patient with an IJ central line in his neck started BLEEDING. I had no idea what to do I just froze. It was the worst feeling. Then my preceptor came in and said let's apply pressure, so we did with some 4X4s. It's just that she was so calm and inside I was freaking out. We ended up transferring him to SDU. Then things just unraveled, we had an empty bed, so we got an ED admit with a pneumothorax and chest tubes just scare me. I was trying to do the admission history but the patient couldn't remember his home meds. Meanwhile my preceptor said we were going to hang blood on another patient. So it didn't get better until almost three o'clock and finally we got to eat.

During your shift, instead of always asking your preceptor what to do, come up with possible solutions. It will make you think harder. Be prepared to offer your rationale. Reading case studies on your own and then discussing them with your preceptor also helps develop critical thinking.

CHAPTER 9

MYTHS OF NURSING PRACTICE

EVIDENCE-BASED PRACTICE

Evidence-based practice is highly important. In fact, the Institute of Medicine has been widely repeated in calling for 90% of clinical decisions to be supported by evidence by 2020.

Strength and Quality

Remember, when citing evidence-based practice, there are different levels of strength of evidence and quality of evidence.

For example, there is no strong clinical evidence around the use of incentive spirometers. Doctors routinely order them, and nurses teach patients to use them.

As quoted by Cochrane, "There is low quality evidence showing a lack of effectiveness of incentive spirometry for prevention of postoperative pulmonary complications in patients after upper abdominal surgery. This review underlines the urgent need to conduct well-designed trials in this field" (do Nascimento Junior P, 2014).

So does that mean incentive spirometers are not helpful? Not necessarily, but it does mean more well-designed randomized clinical studies are needed.

Does that mean they are helpful? Again, the evidence is lacking. What it means is they aren't harmful and may be helpful, but it's not been proven.

Some things are hard to change and one of them is practice myths.

PRACTICE-BASED EVIDENCE

Practice-based evidence is knowledge that comes from experience and practice. Here are some clinical pearls to help you out.

Most of them are practice-based evidence or things I've learned from my own practice, observing patterns and cause and effect.

Best Practice

The other day I heard a clinician state that something was "best practice." I immediately wanted to know what she meant.

Best practice can be based on evidence, or it can be an expert opinion, conventional wisdom, or what has come to be practice based on prestigious or highly regarded clinicians or organizations recommending it. So when someone tells you it is best practice, it is okay to ask for the source. Sometimes it just means it's their opinion and how they want something done.

Anecdotal Practice

Many nursing interventions exist not because there is evidence for their use, but because the interventions have become routine in the absence of clinical data. In other words, some things are done because "we've always done it this way." (Also see the entry on "Evidence-Based Practice" in Chapter 6: Pro Tips A–Z).

It's not just nurses, either. Doctors will vary their practice from the norm based on their personal experiences. Once an orthopedic surgeon had a patient whose hip dislocated while sitting in a chair. Now all his order sets include a personalized order: "No sitting in chair." It doesn't matter if the patient can be placed in a chair that adjusts so the patient is never at 90 degrees—his patients never sit in chairs. It does change usual practice for nurses and PT when mobilizing his patients. His patients sit on the edge of the bed for meals.

As a newly licensed nurse, you will be subject to other nurses, even experienced nurses, giving you incorrect and outdated information. It may have been what they were taught. When a clinician insists on a practice that contradicts what you've been taught, have confidence and ask, "I would love to read more about that, can you share the source for that?" They probably won't be able to. In reality, as a newly graduated nurse, you have recently been given the latest guidelines and best practice.

It's not a defense to say "someone else" told you to do thus-and-so. You are responsible for your own nursing practice.

INFLATING FOLEY BALLOON TO TEST PRIOR TO INSERTION

Inflating the balloon can cause micro trauma from creasing of the silicone balloon. The manufacturer has quality assurance (QA) processes in place. The product works, it doesn't need to be tested.

Don't do it, even if it's hard to resist inflating the balloon.

NPO BEFORE SURGERY

Despite the lack of scientific data, the practice has been that patients had to fast for long intervals before surgery or procedures to avoid aspiration. In many areas, patients are still instructed to refrain from food or drink starting at midnight before surgery. Essentially, they are fasting. Many hospitals still hold to this regime despite the fact there is a risk of dehydration or hypoglycemia from prolonged fasting and of cases being delayed which causes prolonged fasting.

The American Society of Anesthesiologists (ASA) released guidelines around perioperative fasting many years ago:

For healthy patients:
- A meal may be eaten eight hours prior to surgery
- A light meal may be eaten six hours prior to surgery
- Clear liquids may be given up to two hours before surgery

For infants:
- Formula or nonhuman milk may be given six hours prior to surgery
- Breast Milk may be given up to four hours before surgery

Additional fasting time (*e.g.*, eight or more hours) may be needed in cases of patient intake of fried foods, fatty foods, or meat, and clear liquids should not include alcohol.

Pre-operative good nutrition is linked to improved surgical outcomes. Insulin resistance is a known result of fasting, and while not in the ASA Guidelines, there is a theory that carbohydrate loading via carbohydrate clear liquid drinks before surgery is a benefit.

PROTECTIVE ISOLATION

There's a lack of consensus and standardization around the use of protective isolation, sometimes called reverse isolation, or neutropenic isolation. Protective isolation was eliminated as an isolation by the CDC years ago because the evidence does not show that it benefits patients with leukopenia. (Neutropenic precautions are not a form of isolation; they are precautions).

There are three kinds of isolation: contact, airborne, and droplet. That is why you most likely have standardized door signs for contact isolation, airborne isolation, and droplet isolation, but you cannot find a similar door sign for Protective Isolation.

For patients receiving chemotherapy, previous standard practice was to place the patient in protective/reverse isolation. The literature tells us that isolation is difficult for patients and makes them feel, well, isolated and untouchable. The Oncology Nurses Society (ONS) recommends avoiding fresh fruit, live plants, and visitors with colds, but not protective/reverse isolation. The CDC and the ONS both recommend not allowing fresh flowers or plants for immunocompromised patients. Remember that an apple can be washed, a banana and orange peeled, so they're okay. Most hospitals don't serve fresh fruit, anyway. Visitors with colds should stay away.

The problem is that some doctors and some nurses still insist on protective/reverse isolation. If some nurses do not practice protective isolation because they are following evidence-based criteria, but some nurses do routinely mask, gloves, and gown for oncology patients, this leaves the patient and family confused and wondering if the hospital really knows what it's doing.

Lynda's thirty-eight-year-old husband was admitted repeatedly with complications from Hodgkin's lymphoma. Some of the nurses wore masks when entering the room, as did the doctor. Some nursing assistants wore masks, gowns, and gloves. Some nurses wore nothing. One day I was on the unit and Lynda stepped into the hall, wearing a mask and gloves. She said loudly, "Does anyone know what they're doing here? Everyone tells me something different about what I'm supposed to do to protect my husband, even my doctor!" She then burst into tears.

It was very distressful to see her so upset. It was even more distressful to know that we had caused the confusion by our inconsistent practice and patient education. Another good reason for us all to be on the same page and practice evidence-based medicine.

Protective Precautions

There is an isolation called protective precautions. The CDC recommends protective precautions should be used for patients receiving hematopoietic stem cell transplants.

Always remember the single most important measure to prevent infection is hand washing.

SANDBAGS APPLIED TO FEMORAL ARTERY SITE AFTER SHEATH PULL TO CONTROL BLEEDING

Some doctors and nurses place a five-pound sandbag on the femoral artery insertion site after hemostasis is achieved in a femoral sheath pull. There is no evidence that a sandbag will prevent or stop arterial bleeds, and it obscures the view of the puncture site by the nurse when assessing.

Evidence does not support the use of sandbags as a compression method to decrease vascular complications or discomfort. A sandbag exerts diffuse pressure and will definitely not stop an arterial bleed! Some MDs order sandbags to be applied after hemostasis. It won't hurt anything, but be careful it doesn't give you a false sense of security about preventing or controlling bleeding.

There is a plus—it may remind your patient not to flex their affected extremity.

Ruben's patient started bleeding from the site in her neck where a jugular catheter had just been removed. She was bleeding quite profusely and Ruben applied a bulky pressure dressing. Worse, Ruben had an orientee with him.

Did it work? I asked later, knowing the answer. No, it did not work. Manual pressure stops bleeding, not dressings or sandbags. Hold until it clots off.

STAT GLUCOSE TO VERIFY HYPOGLYCEMIA

Some nurses want to "verify" abnormally low glucometer results by ordering a stat lab glucose. But if your patient is symptomatic, you will follow your hospital protocol and immediately administer oral carbs or push D50. By the time lab arrives to draw a stat lab, your patient has been treated. Whatever their blood sugar is now, it can't be used to "verify" your previous result. (Some protocols include performing a second fingerstick test to compare to the first reading.)

If the rationale is to "verify" glucometer readings before treating a patient, then the underlying assumption is that the machine is inaccurate. In which case why are we using it? The opposite assumption is actually the correct one. Point of care glucometer testing is accurate unless proven otherwise.

Of course, always follow your hospital's policy, but always be a critical thinker as well.

TRENDELENBURG FOR SHOCK AND HYPOTENSION

Weak evidence exists for this time-honored intervention, and you may panic trying to remember how to quickly put a bed into Trendelenburg. Current data to support the use of the Trendelenburg position during shock are limited and do not reveal any beneficial or sustained changes in systolic blood pressure or cardiac output. Some deleterious effects have been documented.

Trendelenburg is no longer recommended for shock and hypotension and instead places patients at risk for hemo-dynamic compromise and increased intracranial pressure. Trendelenburg does not lead to improved cardiac output.

TUBE FEEDINGS AND CHECKING GASTRIC RESIDUAL VOLUMES

Historically, tube feedings are stopped for gastric residual volumes of anywhere from 200mL–250mL, and gastric residual volumes are checked every two to four hours. This was due to a fear of aspiration leading to pneumonia. This practice has changed with the goal being to increase nutritional volume. The literature now shows that there is no strong evidence between aspiration pneumonia and GRV (Boullata, J., et al p.86).

Gastric Residual Volume and Risk of Aspiration

Due to the above practice of relying on GRV, too many patients received too little nutrition, with the volume delivered falling far short of the volume ordered. Goal feeding rates were never achieved. This puts patients at risk of nutritional insufficiency. Instead, evaluate patient tolerance to tube feeding using the following:

- Subjective complaints
- Physical exam (abdominal distention)
- Objective findings (gastric residual volume, diarrhea, vomiting)

According to Boullata, J., et al. (p.86) in "ASPEN Safe Practices for Enteral Nutrition Therapy," "GRV measurements may not need to be used as part of routine care to monitor ICU patients on EN. For those patient care areas where GRVs are still utilized, holding EN for GRVs (less than) 500 mL in the absence of other signs of intolerance should be avoided. A gastric residual volume of between 250 and 500 mL should lead to implementation of measures to reduce risk of aspiration."

Interrupting Enteral Tube Feedings and Risk of Aspiration

The head of the bed should be elevated at least thirty degrees (thirty degrees for non-ventilated patients, forty-five for ventilated patients since forty-five degrees is recommended to prevent ventilator-associated pneumonia.) Interrupting the feeding to reposition the patient for a short period of time is not recommended.

PATIENT ABANDONMENT

You may hear conflicting explanations of what constitutes patient abandonment.

> Annette works in a long-term care facility with chronic staffing issues. She showed up to work and clocked in only to find out she was going to be assigned one entire hall of thirty-two patients because another nurse had called in. This was not the first time, and the last time it happened to her, she vowed never to work under such conditions again. She said, "No way," clocked out and left. The DON texted her and said, "I'm reporting you to the BON for patient abandonment unless you get back here ASAP, Annette."

Did Annette abandon her patients? No. She had no patients to abandon. To abandon a patient, a nurse-patient relationship must have been established. The relationship starts when the nurse accepts responsibility for care of the patient. If Annette had received hand-off report, the nurse-patient relationship would have been established. What Annette did was abandon her job, not her patients. She could be fired, but not lose her license.

Note that the BON does not have jurisdiction over employer-employee relationships. So Annette can be fired as her employer sees fit.

Once the nurse-patient relationship has been established, the nurse cannot leave until she, in turn, gives handoff report to another qualified nurse, or the patient is transferred, dies, or is discharged. In this case, Annette never assumed a patient assignment and never took over care of any of the patients. Was Annette's behavior professional? No, of course not. But it was not patient abandonment.

What is Considered Patient Abandonment?

- Failure to notify the employer when you won't be going to work (No-call, No-show) is not patient abandonment.
- Showing up to work and leaving before accepting responsibility for the care of patients is not patient abandonment.
- Refusing a patient assignment is not abandonment. Maybe you lack the skill or knowledge to provide competent care. An example would be a med-surg nurse refusing a NICU assignment, or the care of a continuous renal replacement therapy (CRRT) patient in ICU without oversight.
- Severing the nurse-patient relationship once you have accepted responsibility of the patient without reasonable notice to the appropriate person (typically a supervisor) so arrangements can be made for continuation of nursing care by others is patient abandonment and can lead to discipline by the BON.
- Sleeping on duty (while on the clock) can be considered abandonment.
- Refusing mandatory overtime is not abandonment of patient but nuances of mandatory overtime laws vary state-to-state.

The CA BRN website states: "A nurse–patient relationship begins when responsibility for nursing care of a patient is accepted by the nurse. Failure to notify the employing agency that the nurse will not appear to work an assigned shift is not considered patient abandonment by the BRN, nor is refusal to accept an assignment considered patient abandonment. Once the nurse has accepted responsibility for nursing care of a patient, severing of the nurse–patient relationship without reasonable notice may lead to discipline of a nurse's license."

OVERTIME

Currently, mandatory overtime has been banned in nineteen states with exceptions for emergencies. Normal work hours are considered twelve hours or less.

States Where Mandatory Overtime Has Been Banned

- Alaska
- California
- Connecticut
- Illinois
- Maine
- Maryland
- Massachusetts
- Minnesota
- Missouri
- New Hampshire
- New Jersey
- New York
- Ohio
- Oregon
- Pennsylvania
- Rhode Island
- Texas
- Washington
- West Virginia

Even if your state allows mandatory overtime, some states prohibit employers from taking negative action against a nurse who refuses to stay after a shift to work more hours (Minnesota). You can see that it's very important to find out the laws on mandatory overtime in your state.

When a Nurse is Fatigued
Fatigued nurses have a diminished ability to deliver safe care. The RN must exercise critical judgment regarding their individual ability to practice safe nursing when asked to work overtime. Refusing to work extra hours or shifts because of fatigue is not considered patient abandonment by the BON/BRN. However, it should be noted that the BON/BRN has no jurisdiction over employment and contracts.

TWO DOCTORS SIGNING EMERGENCY CONSENT

If the patient is unable to give informed consent—for example, if the patient is unresponsive or confused—and there are no surrogate decision makers present, the provider need only document that it is an emergency. If the procedure is needed to prevent death, alleviate severe pain, or prevent permanent disability, the provider must document a note, but a consent is not signed.

A doctor never signs a patient consent, much less two doctors.

VASELINE OR OCCLUSIVE DRESSING FOR DISLODGED CHEST TUBE

Use a sterile gauze dressing taped on three corners only in the event of a chest tube dislodgement. An occlusive dressing can cause a tension pneumothorax in a patient with a pneumothorax.

WET TO DRY DRESSING CHANGES

Wet to dry dressing changes are when gauze is soaked (usually in normal saline), placed or packed in the wound bed, and covered with dry gauze. At the next dressing change, the gauze previously soaked in saline has now dried and it is removed, ripping debris but also viable tissue along with it. It was used as a method of debridement. This is very painful for the patient. It used to be thought that ripping off the granulation tissue underneath when changing the dressing stimulated healing and growth.

While preserving an optimally moist wound bed is now recognized as one of the key factors in wound healing and in producing desired outcomes, wet-to-dry gauze dressings do not assure a moist wound.

Moist dressings and wet-to-dry dressings should not be confused. In actuality disturbing the wound bed as described above results in vasoconstriction and injured tissue.

Gauze used to be the only choice for dressing a wound, but gauze has serious drawbacks. Other products are far better for wound granulation than gauze.

Doctors ordering wet-to-dry dressings may be ordering them out of habit and not deliberate choice. Suggest a wound consult. You will find that in certain areas, nurses are far more up-to-date with evidence-based wound management than doctors. With the advent of foams, hydrogels, and alginates, wound care is a nursing specialty of its own. Many doctors (and nurses) have little interest in the nuances of wound care and are happy to have an expert wound care specialist take over.

CHAPTER 10

DISCIPLINARY PROCESS

SIGNS OF TROUBLE

There's been a change in how your preceptor responds to you. Your preceptor seems less patient and makes less eye contact, which is an advanced sign.

What do these signs mean? Most likely there's a performance discrepancy of some kind. They may feel they've told you something repeatedly and you have not changed your behavior.

Time Management

If your preceptor or manager says, "You need to improve your time management," it usually means they expect you to speed up. This is common for all new grads and sometimes it's also unrealistic. You cannot be compared to a nurse who's been practicing for years. If you feel you are doing well with your time management and need to clarify, thank her for the feedback and ask, "How specifically would it look if my time management improved?" This prompts for measurable goals such as "completes medication pass in allotted time."

> Paul is a new grad at week twelve in his med-surg orientation. He has been singled out to extend his orientation by two weeks because of his time management skills. He takes a long time passing meds because he looks every medication up and can't seem to differentiate urgent from non-urgent tasks.

Paul needs to change his habits or his performance will not change. Checking medications is important, but on every unit, there are less than fifteen medications that are given frequently, based on the patient population. Once you are familiar with the indications, contraindications, and usual dosages, there is no need to keep looking them up. This suggests anxiety. Paul also needs to develop a sense of urgency for important matters.

Once I watched a nurse passing her 0900 morning medications. Her phone rang, and she picked up. It was the Lab calling to report an abnormally high potassium on one of her patients. She impatiently told the Lab to call back later as she was passing meds, brushing them off. I listened in amazement because she was about to give a potassium supplement to that very patient.

I thought about what would cause a nurse to make this mistake. This nurse had practiced in a skilled nursing facility and perhaps was very task-oriented. Linear thinking just doesn't work in nursing. You constantly have to respond to changing conditions.

The Talk

It's halfway or maybe even further through your orientation, and you haven't received a lot of feedback either way. You think things are going okay, but your manager has called you in for a talk.

You're nervous and have a bad feeling about this. Maybe it's the way she asked. She seemed a bit uncomfortable. You enter and sit down, but she asks you to get up and close the door, please.

Sure enough, she starts with "How's it going?" but soon assumes a "now-let's-be-serious" expression and swiftly segues into "I have some concerns." The concerns are time management and prioritization. What should you do?

Accept Responsibility

When you are given a verbal or written warning or counseling, you are also being given a chance to turns things around and save your job.

It never helps to be defensive when you are being counseled, even when you feel they are wrong or misinformed.

Chances are that your manager hasn't directly observed your performance, but she has received feedback from your coworkers and preceptor. If she says, "It has been brought to my attention" or "Several people say . . .," do not ask who "they" are.

She most likely is not going to divulge names and asking "who" complained may be seen as a way of deflecting or discounting the feedback she's giving.

The best thing is to listen carefully, strive for understanding, and take it to heart.

WHEN YOU ARE BLINDSIDED

The feedback may come as a surprise to you, in which case you can say that you were not aware of these performance problems, but that you appreciate being given the opportunity to (now) improve.

Even if time has passed since a meeting with your manager in which you were taken by surprise, you can remedy an
initially unfavorable reaction by circling back and giving this
message: "I've had some time to think about what you said, and
I see your point."

Ask for Clarification

Make sure you understand exactly what aspect(s) of your performance you are being asked to improve.

Without being defensive or argumentative, ask for clarification.

"I understand that my time management is a problem. How
would my performance look different if my time management
were improved?"

You can also ask for help.

"What do you think would most help me to improve my
prioritization skills?"

SMART GOALS

Your nurse manager should provide you with an action plan. If
not, ask for one! If not a written action plan in so many words,
then be sure you are provided with measurable goals. The best
goals are SMART Goals:

- Specific
- Measurable
- Achievable
- Realistic
- Timely

Your performance goal(s) should include all of the above in
order for you to succeed and for you and your manager both to
know if you've met them.

CLOSE THE LOOP

Ask when you will meet again with her to review your performance. Ask if you can come to her with questions or guidance before that time if needed.

"I'd appreciate frequent feedback from you to see how I'm doing and where I can improve."

This makes the manager a partner and a coach and holds them accountable.

Make a point to stay in close touch informally with short office drop-bys, a smile, a wave. The more closely you stay in contact with your manager, the better.

PRECEPTOR FEEDBACK

Ask your preceptor for at least daily feedback to evaluate your progress.

Informally, at the end of each shift, ask for specific feedback.

"Now, I was working on my time management today, can you give me feedback on how I did?" or "Can you tell me what went well today and what I could have done differently?"

This gives you timely feedback and is also laying the groundwork for your next manager meeting. If your preceptor simply says you did "fine" four shifts in a row, it would be difficult for the manager to refute that, as you have officially received positive performance feedback.

TRANSFER TO ANOTHER UNIT

Sometimes nurses with perceived performance problems are transferred elsewhere as a means of transferring a perceived problem off of their unit.

But sometimes a transfer to a new unit or a different shift can be a good thing. It can provide a fresh start with a new group of coworkers.

Note—In hospitals, organization is hierarchical, meaning it's not good to do an end run around your boss to go higher up. The same goes for complaining to HR. It usually doesn't get the results you want.

CHAPTER 11

PROFESSIONAL DEVELOPMENT

PROPER TITLE

You will see nurses with strings of letters behind their names, and many of these are because they are certified in a specialty. The American Nurses Association (ANA) has provided guidelines for how to list credentials after your name. It comes down to order of importance. Directly after your name, list your highest academic degree, such as BSN or MSN. There is a standard order in which to list your credentials published by the ANA in a position statement in 2009. The purpose was to standardize the listing to increase consumer understanding, ensuring credibility and competency among nurses and consumers alike.

Licensure is mandatory and professional certifications are voluntary and a sign of professional development and expertise.

Order of Credentials

Your credentials should be listed as follows: Highest earned degree, mandated requirements (i.e. licensure), state designations or requirements, national certifications, awards and honors, other certifications.

If you have a BSN or higher, list the BSN first. If you have an MSN, list the MSN but leave off the BSN. While an Associate Degree in Nursing (ADN) may be included in your resume, don't include it after your name. List the credentials as capital letters without periods between letters. Place a comma between each credential.

Example:
Laura Knowles, MSN, RN, CCRN. Do not write Laura Knowles, BSN, MSN, RN, CCRN as you list only the highest academic credential.

Associate Degree in Nursing (ADN), Bachelor of Science Degree in Nursing (BSN), Master of Science Degree in Nursing, and Doctorate in Nursing (PhD and DNP), are all academic college degrees.

All nurses take the NCLEX for RN licensure. The NCLEX is the same regardless of educational preparation.

ACADEMIC DEGREES

Associate Degree in Nursing (ADN)
ADN degrees are offered by community colleges and vocational schools. Nurses with an ADN complete a two-year program after completing prerequisites such as Anatomy, Physiology, and Chemistry.

ADN prepares nurses for clinical bedside practice but does not prepare nurses for non-clinical roles. An ADN is a great start that gives people the opportunity to get into nursing and from there further their education.

Bachelor of Science Degree in Nursing (BSN)

BSN degrees are offered by four-year colleges. It's important to note that employers are increasingly requiring a BSN or plans to obtain a BSN within a specified time frame. Opportunities for advancement are severely limited by not having a BSN.

Nurses with an ADN degree can enroll in online BSN programs, expecting that there may be some clinical hours required, in which case you will have to arrange for a preceptor. Your organization will need to have an affiliate agreement with your school, and it may be up to you to ask a qualified nurse to serve as your preceptor.

Master of Science Degree in Nursing (MSN)

The difference between a bachelor's degree and a master's degree is narrowing of focus. You have to earn your bachelor's as a pre-requisite to earning your master's, unless it's a direct-entry program. In a bachelor's program, every student takes the same courses. In a master's program, everyone takes the same core classes to start with, then branches off to their area of interest and study.

There are many online MSN programs. Nurses who hold a clinical master's degree are called advanced practice registered nurses (APRNs). MSN programs take between eighteen and twenty-four months, and job growth is projected to be 31% for APRNs from 2012 to 2022. There are many examples of advanced practice nurses:

- Nurse Practitioner (NP)
- Certified Nurse Midwives
- Certified Registered Nurse Anesthetist (CRNAs)

You can earn a master's degree in education, informatics, nursing administration, and more.

Doctorate of Nursing

A doctoral degree is the terminal degree in nursing. There are two types of doctorates. Both are scholarly degrees.

PhD: A PhD in nursing prepares nurses to conduct research to advance the practice of nursing.

DNP: A Doctorate in Nursing Practice prepares nurses to practice nursing at the highest level. APRNs can go on to obtain their DNP. It is predicted that at some point in the future, APRNs will be required to hold a doctorate degree.

A doctoral degree takes three to five years and most often is done by nurses who are working in their area of interest while pursuing their degree.

I hope this helps with deciphering college-speak for college students and nurses of all levels.

CERTIFICATES AND CERTIFICATIONS

There is a difference between certificates and certifications, and it can be confusing. Earning a certificate is not the same as becoming certified.

Certificates

Examples of certificates that are not certifications

> Ashley works on a med-surg oncology unit and was prompted by her nurse manager to obtain her ONS chemotherapy and biotherapy provider certificate. Nurses on the unit need the certificate before they can administer chemotherapy. She earned a certificate but is not a certified nurse.

Nurses who work on oncology units may complete the ONS provider course. At the end of the course, the student is awarded a certificate as a provider of chemotherapy and immunotherapy. This does not allow Ashley to put any credentials behind her name as she is not certified in the specialty of oncology; she earned a certificate saying she can administer chemo medications.

Think of it as a BLS provider card. Likewise, passing an Arrhythmia competency at one hospital may confer an internal certificate, but know that this certificate is home grown and has little value outside of the organization. There is no standardized Arrhythmia exam. At every hospital you work for, you will be required to demonstrate competency in arrhythmia.

Certifications

Most certifications require a substantial number of clinical hours, although there are exceptions. The SCRN certification requires just one year of practice as an RN with direct or indirect stroke nursing experience.

Certification as an oncology nurses is the ONC, a certification offered by ONS. Eligibility requires one thousand clinical hours in oncology. To put it into context, a full-time nurse working twelve-hour shifts works 1,872 hours per year. A full-time nurse working eight-hour shifts works 2,080 hours per year.

Several examples of common certifications in nursing specialties are listed at the end of this chapter. For example, an ICU nurse may choose to earn their CCRN. In that case, their title would be Ashley Brown, BSN, RN, CCRN.

Buyer Beware

Recently Maria came in to take her Arrhythmia exam after completing a course and being awarded a certificate by a company I'll call Questionable.com. She spent $150 and passed her exam with a score of 85%. She took our test and achieved

20%. Who knows what criteria company Questionable.com used. There is no oversight, so anyone who wants to teach a course, charge money, and issue a certificate can do so.

Puzzled at her poor results, I asked Maria to explain her answer of SVT on a strip that was clearly a-fib. She said they did not cover atrial fibrillation and she was unfamiliar with the term.

Likewise, take CPR from the American Heart Association (AHA) only. As a healthcare provider, you are required to hold a current healthcare provider certificate, not a non-healthcare certificate. A red flag is companies that offer online only CPR certificates. AHA requires validation of compressions and breathing, which cannot be done online.

RESUME

Keep your resume updated. When you apply to another job down the road you will need to organize your resume for the individual organization, but if you keep it updated as you go, it will be so much easier.

Keep your list of accomplishments on your resume current. For example, if your facility trained you on customer service such as Studer Group AIDET training, include this training on your resume. In today's market with an emphasis on patient satisfaction, it will be noticed.

If you participated in a unit based council, Shared Governance, or other committees, include them. Take credit for any performance improvement initiatives you or your unit participated in.

PRO-NURSING LANGUAGE

Ever notice how job titles change? Environmental Services used to be called Housekeeping. X-ray Department is now called Diagnostic Imaging. Often these are done to be more descriptive and to elevate the title.

Language is important. It's so important because words change our brains. The Academy of Medical-Surgical Nurses (AMSN) published pro-nursing language to change the way nursing is perceived. Instead of saying, "work on the floor," or "floor nurse/staff nurse," say "practice on the unit" and "clinical nurse." Instead of calling new graduate nurses "newbies" or "babies," use the term "newly licensed nurses."

CONTINUING EDUCATION

Tiffany's license was due to expire at the end of the month. Two weeks before the expiration date, she tallied up her hours on her accumulated certificates, and she realized she was ten contact hours short of the required thirty.

On closer inspection, a certificate she received from a nursing conference was missing the provider number. Would it be accepted? (It would not be accepted). The certificate said "six contact hours" but there was no provider number at the bottom of the certificate. Tiffany panicked and began to frantically search for online courses.

The certificate Tiffany questioned had a topic titled "Management of the Diabetic Patient." It listed six contact hours, but there was no provider number at the bottom. Now she was another six hours short of her required thrity contact hours. Providers of continuing education must include their provider number on the certificate. Provider numbers are issued by approvers.

Approved Providers

Contact hours must be obtained from an approved provider. What is meant by approved provider?

CE providers must be approved by your state's BON/BRN or by the American Nurses Credentialing Center (ANCC). ANCC-approved providers are considered the gold standard. Every BON/BRN accepts courses offered by a provider approved by the ANCC.

For example, national nursing organizations that provide CEs at annual conventions are approved by the ANCC. This is so that nurses from all states can earn CEs at the conference that will be accepted by individual state BON/BRNs.

Some state boards of nursing also approve providers of continuing nursing education activities. Your hospital may have applied to the state board of nursing to be a provider and would then have been issued a provider number.

Another very important thing to look for besides a provider number is that the provider is recognized by *your* state board of nursing. For example, a provider approved by the Florida Board of Nursing is not recognized by the California Board of Registered Nurses.

Let's say a nurse in California attended an educational event in Florida. They are given a certificate for five hours with a provider number. It also says approved by the Florida State Board of Nursing. They will not be able to use this continuing education when renewing their California license.

DIFFERENCE BETWEEN CEUs, CONTACT HOURS, AND CEs

- CE refers to continuing education. Continuing nursing education is CNE. CE and CNE, used interchangeably, are not a measure of time or credit.

- Contact hours is a measure that represents an hour of scheduled instruction given to a student. The term "contact hour" is used by the American Nurses Credentialing Center (ANCC) and is fifty or sixty minutes of instruction in a board-approved nursing continuing education class or activity.
- CEU refers to a continuing education unit. One CEU equals ten contact hours.

The terms CEU and CE are often used interchangeably with contact hours as in "I earned four CEUs (or CEs)." This is a mistake when the correct language is "I earned four contact hours."

LICENSING RENEWAL AND CONTINUING EDUCATION REQUIREMENTS BY STATE

Continuing education requirements vary from state to state and are governed by the state Board of Nursing or state Board of Registered Nursing. Be sure to see your state Board of Nursing or Board of Registered Nursing's website for requirements. You can visit the National Council State Boards of Nursing (NCSBN) website at www.ncsbn.org for more information.

Many states waive continuing education for a newly licensed nurse for their first renewal period. In addition to continuing education requirements varying by state, license renewal time varies. Many states require license renewal every two years, but some require it annually and some every three years.

Continuing education may not be earned and saved ahead of time; it must be obtained within the renewal period preceding the license renewal date. As an example, if a nurse resides in a state that renews biennially and is required to renew his or her license by July 31, 2023, then the CE requirements must have been completed between August 1, 2021, and July 31, 2023.

State Variance

In addition to requiring a certain number of contact hours for license renewal, some states have specific continuing educational requirements related to particular clinical topics. As an example, Nevada has a one-time requirement for four hours of bioterrorism education. New Jersey requires one hour on prescription opioids and Florida has a long list of requirements:

- Two hours related to medical error prevention each renewal;
- Two hours on the laws and rules that govern the practice of nursing in Florida;
- One hour related to HIV/AIDS;
- Two hours related to recognizing impairment in the workplace every four years; and for each third renewal period, an additional two hours related to domestic violence.

California requires thirty contact hours every two years, but Arizona requires none. North Carolina requires fifteen contact hours and 640 hours of practice. Rhode Island requires ten contact hours, two of which must be on substance abuse. Kentucky nurses must renew their license every year, and Arizona is every four years with no continuing education requirements.

Jenny moved to California after having worked in Arizona for years, endorsing her license to California. Arizona has no continuing education requirements. California requires thirty contact hours every two years. Jenny forgot California's requirement and came close to not meeting her continuing education requirements and not being eligible for re-licensure.

Some states will accept alternate methods of meeting continuing education requirements. A national certification in a nursing specialty or publication in a peer-reviewed journal may be accepted.

Criteria for Continuing Education Content

Not everything is considered acceptable content for CE credit. Typically, CE must be relevant to the nursing practice and augment basic nursing knowledge. When you are advancing your education through an accredited BSN or graduate degree program, your academic units count for CNE credit. General education courses do not count for CNE credit.

Typically, one academic semester unit is equal to fifteen contact hours; one academic quarter unit is equal to ten contact hours.

Courses Not Accepted

Prerequisite courses, such as mathematics, government, anatomy, physiology, and general education courses are not accepted as CNE credit.

Advanced Skills Renewal Courses such as Advanced Cardiac Life Support (ACLS) and Pediatric Advanced Life Support (PALS) may be counted when they are initially obtained but not by every state when they are renewed. Check your state's requirements.

Hours spent in new hire Orientation do not count. Self-improvement courses that focus on changes in attitude, self-improvement, weight loss, or yoga are typically not accepted.

In some states (for example, CA) nurses may use Category I continuing medical education (CMEs) such as those offered at vendor-sponsored educational activities for medical providers, but in other states, only advanced practice registered nurses (APRNs) may use CMEs.

The following activities are more examples of activities that are not acceptable for CE credit in most states:

- Basic CPR
- On-the-job training and equipment demonstration
- Refresher courses designed to update knowledge
- Orientation programs designed to introduce employees to a specific work setting
- Economic courses for financial gain, e.g., investments, retirement, preparing resumes, and techniques for job interviews
- Liberal Arts courses in music, art, philosophy, etc. when unrelated to patient/client care
- Courses designed for lay people
- Repetition of any educational activity with identical content and objectives within a single reporting period
- Agency-specific orientation or in-service programs
- Self-directed independent study activities that have not been approved for CE
- Community service or volunteer practice
- Administrative or disciplinary CE
- Membership in a professional nursing organization
- Professional meetings or conventions except for those portions approved for CE

Meaningful Education

Many nurses wait until the last minute to earn CEs and choose topics based on price or on a prediction of how easy it will be to pass the course. In order to keep pace with the rapidly changing healthcare environment, the BON/BRN expects each licensee to maintain and improve competencies in current knowledge, skills, and abilities relevant to area of practice.

Record Keeping
Keep records as if you'll be audited. You'll need title of course taken, number of contact hours awarded, date of course, and provider number. Approved providers are issued a provider number. Scan copies of your certificates to yourself to keep an electronic file. Make sure the certificate has the provider number on it.

How Long to Keep Records
Check with your state BON/BRN. For example, in Texas, nurses must keep continuing education records for three licensure renewal cycles.

Audit Process in Texas:

At least two percent (2%) of the renewal applications will be subject to random audit per renewal cycle. A licensee who submits inaccurate or falsified documentation or fails to meet the CE requirement will be subject to disciplinary action based on Chapter 54-02-07-01.1(7)(13)(18).

Conferences

Manjeet attended a conference the year before but failed to complete and submit his evaluation. He expected the certificate in the mail, but it never came.

Most providers require an evaluation as part of issuing contact hours.

COMPACT LICENSURE

Under the Nurse Licensure Compact (NLC) nurses can practice in compact states without having to obtain additional licensure.

> For example, Carla lives in Texas, which is a compact state, and wants to work in a hospital just across the border in New Mexico, which is also a compact state. Since they are both compact states, Carla can accept a job in New Mexico, or any other compact state, without endorsing her license. Carla cannot accept a job in California, which is a non-compact state, without endorsing to California Board of Registered Nursing.

According to the National Council of State Boards of Nursing (NCSBN) "Only nurses who declare a compact state as their primary state of residence may be eligible for a multistate license. As a resident of a non-compact state, you may apply for a license by endorsement in a compact state. Your eligibility will be limited to a single state license that is valid in that state only. As a resident of a non-compact state, you can have as many single-state licenses as you wish."

This eliminates the time consuming and expensive process of obtaining a single-state license in each state.

The term multistate license is synonymous with compact license. The primary state of residence is not necessarily where you own property. It is the state that issued your driver's license and voter's registration, or the address you use to file federal taxes. The primary state of residence must be a compact state to be eligible for a compact license. A primary state of residence, also called a "home state," is defined by the compact as "the person's fixed, permanent, and principal home for legal purposes" and is generally evidenced by where a nurse holds a driver's license, pays taxes, and/or votes. The nurse must meet requirements for licensure renewal and follow CE requirements for their primary state of residence.

If you hold a license in a state you declared as your primary state of residence and that state is a compact state, you can practice in other compact states under that license. To check if your license is multi-state or single-state, go to www.nursys.com.

CEs and Compact Licensure

The list of states belonging to the Nurse Licensure Compact (NLC) is located on the web page for the National Council of State Boards of Nursing: www.ncsbn.org/nlc.htm.

The NLC facilitates nursing practice among states without requiring additional licensure. State barriers are breaking down with the advent of telenursing and telehealth, and travelers move frequently between states.

The NLC grants multi-state privileges and authorizes a nurse licensed and residing in a compact state (home state) to practice in other compact states (remote). The nurse maintains active licensure only in their primary state of residence.

> Jessica's primary state of residence is Colorado, a compact state, where continuing education is not required. Jessica accepts a traveling position in South Dakota, also a compact state, where continuing education is required. Because Jessica's home state is Colorado, she is not required to take continuing education but may practice in South Dakota. Jessica can practice across state lines in all states participating in the compact.

By contrast, if a nurse's home state is Iowa, the nurse must meet Iowa's CE requirements (thirty-six contact hours) even if the nurse only practices in South Dakota (no CE requirements).

Professional Organization Membership

Belonging to your professional organization brings many benefits. You have access to clinical standards of care and evidence-based clinical guidelines and receive a journal membership.

The American Nurses Association is one place to start and the ANA has affiliates in every state. The Association of Women's Health, Obstetric and Neonatal Nurses (AWHONN) is a 501(c)3 membership organization that promotes the health of women & newborns.

Medical-surgical nurses can belong to the Academy of Medical-Surgical Nurses. The professional organization for operative and perioperative nurses is AORN (Association of perioperative Registered Nurses). There is a professional organization for orthopedic nurses and of course the American Association for Critical-Care Nurses (AACN) for critical care nurses.

As a Nursing Professional Development Specialist, I belong to several organizations, including the Infusion Nurses Society (INS) for access to the INS Standards of Care. It's a great resource for looking up all things IV, such as how often to flush an implanted port and how frequently to change IV tubing.

Find a Niche

Learning never stops. I challenge you to find a niche towards the end of your first year. Become an expert on breath sounds and heart sounds. Become an expert on differentiating heart blocks. Start to learn twelve lead EKG skills. Teach yourself all about ABGs.

Networking

Networking is not just for experienced nurses and non-bedside nurses. People with networking skills succeed and the lack of networking skills can hold you back in your career.

Be a Preceptor

You may be asked to serve as a preceptor. You may feel you don't know enough yet to be a preceptor, but you can relate to newly licensed nurses. It will stretch you, but know that preceptors are hand-picked by managers. If you are asked, it is an honor.

Do a self-inventory, as you are now a role model. If you have been taking any shortcuts in practice, now is the time to go back to the right way because a newly licensed nurse will be looking up to you.

Remember what things you appreciated in your preceptors, and where they could have done better. Praise in public and correct in private. Talk your preceptee up to others—you are their protector, their coach. Remember what it felt like to be a newly licensed nurse.

Continue Your Education

You may be thinking of going back to school to earn your bachelor's or master's degree. You may be looking at becoming a Nurse Practitioner. Education is not only formal education. You may be thinking of changing to another specialty.

CONCLUSION

If you are nearing the end of your first year, congratulations! You are a full-functioning member of the team now. When you see nursing students on the floor, you can look back and realize how far you've come. By now you should no longer feel like a poser and you should feel comfortable in your own skin as a clinician. You should no longer have generalized anxiety, but you may still have focused anxiety about complex patient situations.

I hope you realize by now you have chosen the most amazing career in the world. You are only limited by yourself. If you dream it, you can do it. You are marketable! You are most likely fulfilling a contract requirement, but you are no longer and will never again be a newly licensed nurse with no experience.

LIST OF NURSE CERTIFICATIONS

Credentialing Organization	Certification
American Association of Critical Care Nurses Certification Corporation	CCRN Acute Critical Care Nursing PCCN- Progressive Care Nursing (Tele)
American Nurses Credentialing Center	RN-BC Informatics Nursing RN-BC Medical-Surgical Nursing RN-BC Nursing Professional Development RN-BC Nursing Case Management RN-BC Pediatric Nursing
Board of Certification for Emergency Nursing	CEN- Certified Emergency Nurse TCRN- Trauma Certified Registered Nurse
Medical-Surgical Nursing Certification Board	CMSRN Certified Medical-Surgical Registered Nurse
National Certification Corporation	RNC-OB Inpatient Obstetric Nursing RNC-NIC Neonatal Intensive Care Nursing
Oncology Nursing Certification	AOCN Advanced Oncology Certified Nurse
Orthopedic Nurses Certification Board	ONC- Orthopedic Nurse Certified
Pediatric Nursing Certification	CPN Certified Pediatric Nurse
Wound Ostomy and Continence Nursing Certification Board	CWCN Certified Wound Care Nurse CWOCN Certified Wound Ostomy Continence Nurse

CHAPTER 12

JUST FOR FUN

Most nurses have really amazing if not wicked senses of humor. Here are some jokes shared with permission from fellow nurses for no reason whatsoever except to make you laugh. Truth is stranger than fiction, and you just can't make this stuff up.

Write down your own funny stories as they happen so you don't forget them.

Patients Say the Darndest Things:

1. A sweet elderly female patient reaches over and pats her doctor's hand. "My, my, you are such a good doctor! Maybe you can be a nurse someday."
2. Elderly female patient being prepped for Cath lab for a coronary angiogram. "I don't know why I'm having this test, dear. I take my Prozac every day, just like my doctor said!"

3. From a nurse with eyes rolled: "My patient's wife told me she's a cardiologist and would like a troponin drawn on her husband here for a hip fracture to see if he has a DVT."

4. My elderly client in an assisted living facility keeps telling me her weight is down to 150 lbs. I asked her again today, "Still down around 150 lbs.?"

   "Yes, 150! When I hold onto the bathroom wall rail. If I let go, it says 195."

5. Nurse to patient after vasectomy, "You can apply a bag of frozen peas to the area when you get home."

   Patient: "But I don't like peas. Can I use corn?"

Co-Workers

1. Doctor with heavy accent is dressed in sterile garb at the bedside in ICU, hands gloved and up in the air, gown on, yelling "Pants! Pants!" Everyone tries to figure out what he wants.

   "Pants!! Pants!!"

   Finally, the nurse comes up behind him, reaches around, unties the drawstring, and yanks his scrub pants down to his ankles in one motion.

   I'm sorry, I never found out what he was really saying but this is a true story as every nurse in my community will attest to. His underwear was jockey style, blue.

2. My officemate, Debbie, when I asked to borrow her stapler, "Sure, but it doesn't work that great. It only staples one page at a time." Ummm . . . okay?

3. I was covering for another nurse who was on her lunch break, and a call light from one of her rooms came on. I was in a particularly good mood that evening and waltzed into the room with a cheerful "WassUp,

homie?" And then I pulled back the curtain . . . and their patient was African-American. I was so embarrassed. It was stupid of me to use the vernacular, anyway. He was okay with it, though." (VivaLasViegas from allnurses. com)

4. Phone rings. New doctor picks up, looks at new nurse ringing him two feet away. Both slide phones back into their pockets.

5. Encouraging Preceptor: "You did a good job taking your weekly wound photos. Now let's take them with the Mepilex off, shall we?"

6. Nurse in pre-op cheerfully says to patient before his below the knee amputation, "We'll have you back up on your feet in no time!"

7. When I was a new student someone asked me to get them a number seven fallopian tube from the supply room cart.

   I must have spent a good 10 minutes looking for that thing. (Pixie from allnurses.com)

8. So the nurse was assisting a doctor who's putting in a femoral line. He said, "Hold the pannus out of the way."

   He looks up. I said, "Hold the PANNUS NOT THE PENIS!"

9. I am not, nor have I ever been, a *complete* idiot. But I have done some truly moronic things. I used to work in a telemetry unit (my first job) where the house staff was divided up into the Red Team and the Blue Team. I had a patient going bad, and the new resident walked into the nurse's station. I wanted to know which team he was on—could I ask him for orders, or would I have to page someone. What I *said* was, "What color are you?"

   The guy looked affronted, and then said, stiffly, "I'm Black."

OMG! I kind of hadn't really noticed—I was looking at the white coat. In my efforts to backpedal, the smartest thing I could come up with to say was, "I can see that. But are you red or blue?"

Fortunately, he saw the humor in my embarrassment, but he never let me forget it.

(Ruby vee from allnurses.com)

10. Tachypnea is better than no pnea at all.

H&Ps

Some H&Ps are hilarious when you have the time to read them.

1. "46 yr. old female appears stated age presents with stomach pain after eating Chinese food at restaurant that also serves fried chicken."
2. As seen in H&P: Pt c/o of passing out and hitting head after drinking. "I woke up unconscious."
3. Reason for visit: Morbidly obese due to excess calories

BIBLIOGRAPHY

CHAPTER 1

Benner, P. (1984). From novice to expert. *Menlo Park.*
Casey K, Fink R, Krugman M, Propst JNurs Adm. 2004 Jun;
  34(6):303-11.
Kramer, M. (1974). *Reality shock; why nurses leave nursing.*
  Mosby.

CHAPTER 2

Patricia Benner, R. N., & Christine Tanner, R. N. (Eds.).
  (2009). *Expertise in nursing practice: Caring, clinical judgment, and ethics.* Springer Publishing Company.
Westrick, S. J. (2013). *Essentials of nursing law and ethics.* Jones
  & Bartlett Publishers.

CHAPTER 3

Geiger-Brown, J., Sagherian, K., Zhu, S., Wieroniey, M. A.,
  Blair, L., Warren, J., . . . Szeles, R. (2016). CE: Original

Research: Napping on the Night Shift: A Two-Hospital Implementation Project. *The American journal of nursing, 116*(5), 26–33. doi:10.1097/01.NAJ.0000482953.88608.80

National Sleep Foundation accessed January, 2016 https:// sleepfoundation.org/sites/default/files/3-Drowsy%20 Driving%20Media%20One%20Sheet-CSG-FINAL.pdf

CHAPTER 4

AACN Standards for establishing and sustaining healthy work environments. Obtained from the web Nov. 2019 https:// www.aacn.org/~/media/aacn-website/nursing-excellence/ healthy-work-environment/execsum.pdf?la=en

Patricia Benner, R. N., & Christine Tanner, R. N. (Eds.). (2009). *Expertise in nursing practice: Caring, clinical judgment, and ethics.* Springer Publishing Company.

CHAPTER 5

Patricia Benner, R. N., & Christine Tanner, R. N. (Eds.). (2009). *Expertise in nursing practice: Caring, clinical judgment, and ethics.* Springer Publishing Company.

Schmalenberg, C., & Kramer, M. (2009). Nurse-physician relationships in hospitals: 20,000 nurses tell their story. *Critical Care Nurse, 29*(1), 74-83.

Stein, L. I. (1967). The doctor-nurse game. *Archives of general psychiatry, 16*(6), 699-703.

CHAPTER 6

Carson, J. L., Guyatt, G., Heddle, N. M., Grossman, B. J., Cohn, C. S., Fung, M. K., ... & Peterson, N. (2016). Clinical practice guidelines from the AABB: red blood cell transfusion thresholds and storage. Jama, 316(19), 2025-2035.

do Nascimento Junior P, Módolo NSP, Andrade S, Guimarães MMF, Braz LG, El Dib R. Incentive spirometry for prevention of postoperative pulmonary complications in upper abdominal surgery. Cochrane Database of Systematic Reviews 2014, Issue 2. Art. No.: CD006058. DOI: 10.1002/14651858.CD006058.pub3

Standard 43. Phlebotomy. Infusion therapy standards of practice. (2016). *Journal of Infusion Nursing, 39,* S84–S88

Juran NB, Rouse CL, Smith DD, O'Brien MA, DeLuca SA, & Sigmon K. (1999). Nursing interventions to decrease bleeding at the femoral access site after percutaneous coronary intervention. *American Journal of Critical Care, 8*(5), 303–313. Retrieved from http://search.ebscohost.com/login.aspx?direct=true&db=ccm&AN=107221850&site=e-host-live

Westrick, S. J. (2013). *Essentials of nursing law and ethics.* Jones & Bartlett Publishers.

CHAPTER 7

Montalvo, I., (September 30, 2007) "The National Database of Nursing Quality Indicators™ (NDNQI®)" OJIN: The Online Journal of Issues in Nursing. Vol. 12 No. 3, Manuscript 2.

The Joint Commission on Accreditation of Healthcare Organizations. *Comprehensive Accreditation Manual for Hospitals.* Glossary. Oakbrook Terrace, IL. 2017 update. (Manual and corresponding updates are subscription-based.)

CHAPTER 8

Alfaro-LeFevre, R. (2015). *Critical Thinking, Clinical Reasoning, and Clinical Judgment E-Book: A Practical Approach.* Elsevier Health Sciences.

Benner, Partricia, R. N., & Christine Tanner, R. N. (Eds.). (2009). *Expertise in nursing practice: Caring, clinical judgment, and ethics.* Springer Publishing Company.

Bittner, N. P., & Tobin, E. (1998). Critical thinking: strategies for clinical practice. *Journal for Nurses in Professional Development, 14*(6), 267-272.

NGN Talks: A Look at the Strategic Practice Analysis and Special Research Section Video Transcript. @2019 National Council State Boards of Nursing. Presenter Novak, Ryan. Accessed via the web July 2019 https://www.ncsbn.org/Transcript_NGNTalk_Episode02.pdf

Papathanasiou, I. V., Kleisiaris, C. F., Fradelos, E. C., Kakou, K., & Kourkouta, L. (2014). Critical thinking: The development of an essential skill for nursing students. *Acta Informatica Medica, 22*(4), 283.

Wenqi Mok, Wenru Wang, Simon Cooper, Emily Neo Kim Ang, Sok Ying Liaw, Attitudes towards vital signs monitoring in the detection of clinical deterioration: scale development and survey of ward nurses, *International Journal for Quality in Health Care*, Volume 27, Issue 3, June 2015, Pages 207–213, https://doi.org/10.1093/intqhc/mzv019

CHAPTER 9

Boullata, J. I., Carrera, A. L., Harvey, L., Escuro, A. A., Hudson, L., Mays, A., . . . & Kinn, T. J. (2017). ASPEN safe practices for enteral nutrition therapy. *Journal of Parenteral and Enteral Nutrition, 41*(1), 15-103.

Bridges, N., & Jarquin-Valdivia, A. A. (2005). Use of the Trendelenburg position as the resuscitation position: to T or not to T?. *American Journal of Critical Care*, *14*(5), 364-368.

McClave, S. A., Taylor, B. E., Martindale, R. G., Warren, M. M., Johnson, D. R., Braunschweig, C., . . . & Gervasio, J. M. (2016). Guidelines for the provision and assessment of nutrition support therapy in the adult critically ill patient: Society of Critical Care Medicine (SCCM) and American Society for Parenteral and Enteral Nutrition (ASPEN). *Journal of Parenteral and Enteral Nutrition*, *40*(2), 159-211.

Juran NB, Rouse CL, Smith DD, O'Brien MA, DeLuca SA, Sigmon K. Nursing interventions to decrease bleeding at the femoral access site after percutaneous coronary intervention. *American Journal of Critical Care*. 1999;8(5):303-313. http://search.ebscohost.com/login.aspx?direct=true&db=ccm&AN=107221850&site=ehost-live. Accessed June 17, 2019.

Pogatschnik, C., & Steiger, E. (2015). Review of preoperative carbohydrate loading. *Nutrition in Clinical Practice*, *30*(5), 660-664.

Practice Guidelines for Preoperative Fasting and the Use of Pharmacologic Agents to Reduce the Risk of Pulmonary Aspiration: Application to Healthy Patients Undergoing Elective Procedures: An Updated Report by the American Society of Anesthesiologists Task Force on Preoperative Fasting and the Use of Pharmacologic Agents to Reduce the Risk of Pulmonary Aspiration*. Anesthesiology 2017;126(3):376-393. doi: 10.1097/ALN.0000000000001452.

Siegel JD, Rhinehart E, Jackson M, Chiarello L, and the Healthcare Infection Control Practices Advisory Committee, 2007 Guideline for Isolation Precautions: Preventing Transmission of Infectious Agents in Healthcare

Settings https://www.cdc.gov/infectioncontrol/guidelines/
isolation/index.html

Winland-Brown, J., Lachman, V. D., & Swanson, E. O. C.
(2015). The new 'Code of ethics for nurses with interpre-
tive statements'(2015): Practical clinical application, Part I.
Medsurg Nursing, 24(4), 268.

Yong, P. L., Saunders, R. S., & Olsen, L. A. (2010). Institute
of Medicine Roundtable on Evidence-Based Medicine.
In *The Healthcare Imperative: Lowering Costs and Improving
Outcomes: Workshop Series Summary (2010)*.